SpringerBriefs in Public Health

SpringerBriefs in Public Health present concise summaries of cutting-edge research and practical applications from across the entire field of public health, with contributions from medicine, bioethics, health economics, public policy, biostatistics, and sociology.

The focus of the series is to highlight current topics in public health of interest to a global audience, including health care policy; social determinants of health; health issues in developing countries; new research methods; chronic and infectious disease epidemics; and innovative health interventions.

Featuring compact volumes of 50 to 125 pages, the series covers a range of content from professional to academic. Possible volumes in the series may consist of timely reports of state-of-the art analytical techniques, reports from the field, snapshots of hot and/or emerging topics, literature reviews, and in-depth case studies. Both solicited and unsolicited manuscripts are considered for publication in this series.

Briefs are published as part of Springer's eBook collection, with millions of users worldwide. In addition, Briefs are available for individual print and electronic purchase.

Briefs are characterized by fast, global electronic dissemination, standard publishing contracts, easy-to-use manuscript preparation and formatting guidelines, and expedited production schedules. We aim for publication 8–12 weeks after acceptance.

Jenny Lieberman

The Physical, Personal, and Social Impact of Spinal Cord Injury

From the Loss of Identity to Achieving a Life Worth Living

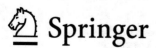 Springer

Jenny Lieberman
Department of Rehabilitation and Human Performance
The Mount Sinai Hospital
New York, NY, USA

ISSN 2192-3698   ISSN 2192-3701   (electronic)
SpringerBriefs in Public Health

ISBN 978-3-031-18651-6   ISBN 978-3-031-18652-3   (eBook)
https://doi.org/10.1007/978-3-031-18652-3

This Springer imprint is published by the registered company Springer Nature Switzerland AG
The registered company address is: Gewerbestrasse 11, 6330 Cham, Switzerland

Preface

John was driving home on a rainy night. Lisa dove into the ocean during spring break and hit the bottom. Sarah was driving a motorcycle in the country and lost control. Alex was hit by a stray bullet while playing in the park. Susan fell from a window. They all sustained a traumatic spinal cord injury. However, each individual's physical outcome and personal experience was different.

A spinal cord injury (SCI) is traumatic and life changing. It impacts the life of the person who has experienced the injury as well as all those in their circle: family, friends, colleagues, lovers, and peers. It is important for all individuals involved to understand what the experience is for the person with SCI and all areas impacted in order to best support the person with SCI, as well as themselves. The goal of this brief is to provide education on all aspects of SCI in hopes of providing clarity. While there is no magical answer in these pages, the contents can provide basic understanding with resources for more specific exploration of information.

This brief explores the many facets of SCI. A SCI impacts each person physically, socially, psychologically, and sometimes cognitively. In order to understand the effect a SCI can have on a person, it is essential to examine all parameters. This brief first explores the physical as a means to provide an understanding of what body changes occur. This remains the most easily understood area in SCI among rehabilitation providers, but is not as easily understood among other healthcare professionals. In order to ensure each individual can live their best life, it is essential all persons involved have a good understanding. From there, this brief goes on to examine what is the subjective meaning and lived experience of disability for persons with SCI. Each individual understands and experiences their disability differently, but there are some themes that are noticeable across all populations of SCI. This is important for family, friends, and healthcare providers to be aware of so they can attempt to understand how each individual experiences this life-altering event. It is also helpful for the person with SCI to have a sense that they are not alone in their response to such a devastating injury. This brief ends with an examination of what organizations and programs exist to promote independence and a sense of community for persons with SCI.

The chapters cover four distinct subjects, each one addressing a different component of SCI. While there is an order in how this brief is designed in discussing the symptoms and experience throughout, feel free to refer to the reference section at the end of each chapter for specific topics. Each chapter also ends with a set of resources to guide the individual with SCI, their family, and their friends in the process.

Chapter 1 explores the objective aspect of SCI. It starts with an overview of SCI, looking at onset and treatment. Statistics and literature are used to examine incidence of injury, healthcare utilization, barriers to healthcare, and educational and employment opportunities.

Chapter 2 highlights the rehabilitation process, examining all stages of rehabilitation, the multi-disciplinary team, and various technologies that can promote improved function and independence. Rehabilitation plays an important role in the pursuit of a meaningful life by teaching the person with SCI what is possible with their body and how to become more independent.

Chapter 3 looks at existing phenomenological and narrative research to subjectively explore the experience and meaning for the individual. Considerations for support and recovery are presented to glean how the person with SCI might be experiencing their changed life, identifying ways people and organizations can aid in the transition into societal reentry.

The final chapter of this book (Chap. 4) examines academic and economic opportunities. There are various consequences of disability that interfere in the ability to participate in academic programs or in acquisition of employment prospects. These are explored in great length, with factors ranging from societal bias to familial factors to governmental programs. Finances play a large role in the opportunity for success in SCI. In urban areas, the primary cause of SCI is violence. The residences are apartments. And sometimes, the only point of discharge is a nursing home. With changes in insurance reimbursement, length of stay has decreased. The result is young men and women, who cannot yet emotionally process what has happened to them, are being forced to learn how to live in their changed bodies. The dilemma is promoting the sense of a life worth living in an unknown body. This makes access to programs even more valuable.

New York, NY, USA   Jenny Lieberman

Acknowledgments

This completed brief could not have been possible without the support of many individuals. First, I wish to thank my Mom and Dad for their unconditional love and constant support. To my friends with spinal cord injury, and to those who I have worked with over the past 25 years, thank you for trusting me and for teaching me. You are the reason I am writing this brief. To Marc Skalias, with love. Thank you for your patience through all the ups and downs. I couldn't have done this without you. Finally, I wish to dedicate this brief to Kenneth Gant, for introducing me to wheelchair seating and positioning, and to Jim Hinojosa for making me believe I could write anything. I wish I could share this with you.

Contents

About the Author

Jenny Lieberman PhD, OTR/L, ATP, is a senior clinical specialist of wheelchair seating and positioning in the Department of Rehabilitation and Human Performance at The Mount Sinai Hospital Center in New York, NY, USA. She is also an adjunct professor in the Department of Occupational Therapy at New York University in New York, NY, USA.

Chapter 1
Background

Spinal cord injury (SCI) can be due to a traumatic event, vascular change, inflammatory process, or malignancy. The most common cause of SCI is trauma. A traumatic SCI occurs when there is a sudden or traumatic blow to the spinal cord that is either a direct tearing of tissue (i.e., a bullet, shattered bone, or sharp object) or dislocation of vertebrae. Damage occurs at the moment of impact when bony fragments or disk material contact the spine, causing either tearing of the cord or bruising. A complete severing of the cord is less common than damage of the nerves of the spinal column. This can present itself as trauma to almost all the nerves or just a small area. For this reason, neurological recovery can never truly be pictured until tissue healing occurs.

Though direct trauma is the leading cause of SCI, there are several diagnoses that can result in SCI, with the same presentation and outcome. Infection, inflammation, vascular events, and degenerative orthopedic changes can all impact the spine and cause permanent trauma.

Spondylosis is a condition that results in degeneration of intervertebral disks over time. On occasion, this can result in compression on the spinal cord and nerve roots. This can result in loss of motor function, sensation, and even bladder and bowel function.

Transverse myelitis is an inflammation that affects a portion of the spinal cord. It can occur at any level, damaging the myelin (the tissue that covers nerve fibers) and interrupting nerve transmission. Causes can be infection or an immune system disorder. Recovery can occur within the first 3 months to 2 years. However, if there is no improvement in the first 6 months, full recovery is unlikely.

Spinal strokes can occur from hemorrhage (bleeding) or ischemia (a blood clot) to the blood supply along the spinal cord. There are many vessels, with the anterior vertebral artery most frequently being the one affected. When this occurs, there is often tissue death that results in subsequent nervous system dysfunction.

Tumors in the spine are another cause of SCI. Whether a solid mass or an invasive growth into vascular and nerve tissue, intervention determines the outcome.

© The Author(s) 2022
J. Lieberman, *The Physical, Personal, and Social Impact of Spinal Cord Injury*,
SpringerBriefs in Public Health, https://doi.org/10.1007/978-3-031-18652-3_1

Surgical removal can sometime result in the necessary removal of healthy tissue to ensure acquiring all malignant tissue.

1.1 Anatomy

The spine consists of bones, one stacked upon the other, running from the base of the skull to the pelvis. The spine contains vertebrae, which provide protection to the spinal cord. Nerves exit at each vertebrae, traveling to various muscles, sensory points, and organs. The pathway for transferring information from the brain to the muscles, skin, and organs can be interrupted at any point. This interruption can be caused by a direct tearing or ripping of nerves, resulting in trauma to the surrounding area and inflammation.

The spinal cord consists of five separate regions: cervical, thoracic, lumbar, sacral, and coccyx. The location of injury determines neurological involvement, with the higher up the injury, the greater potential for impact on the entire body as well as physiological function (breathing, swallowing, and elimination). There are 31 pairs of spinal nerves exiting the spinal cord. The nerves affecting motor exit from the front of the spinal cord, while those that affect sensation exit from the back. This includes touch and pressure, pain, temperature, and body position. These nerves receive and distribute information (Figs. 1.1, 1.2, and 1.3).

It is important to understand that due to the complex nature of nerve configuration and anatomy, not all injuries are the same. Some injuries can result in complete loss of motor and sensory function, while others impact one function or the other. Some injuries result in partial loss of either as well. The spinal cord has a universal layout in regard to pathways, but anatomical anomalies can occur. However, having an understanding of the location of injury can assist in generalizing physical outcome (Fig. 1.4).

Each level of the spine correlates to a different portion of the body. Cervical spine injuries (C1–C8) result in tetraplegia. The higher the level, the greater the impact on physiological function. Injuries above C4 often impact respiration and can result in the need for a ventilator to assist breathing. Shoulder movements and elbow flexion occur at C6, with elbow and wrist extension at C7. C6/C7 is a key area for function due to the onset of tenodesis. Tenodesis is a movement pattern that automatically pulls down the finger flexors when the wrist extends, allowing for grasp and pinch. While not a true grasp or pinch, this movement pattern allows for greater independence in all areas of self-care. Finger movements develop at C8. As long as the cervical spine is impacted, there is some level of upper extremity involvement. Prehension and hand function remain impacted between C7 and sometimes T1 depending on individual anatomy.

Thoracic level injuries result in paraplegia. The vertebrae in this level are T1 to T12. Injuries between T1 and T8 impact the abdominal and thoracic wall and can affect respiratory capacity and trunk control. The absence of muscles here impacts the ability to inhale deeply or sit unsupported. Injuries between T9 and T12 result in

Fig. 1.1 Spinal cord front
view; Mimi Smith

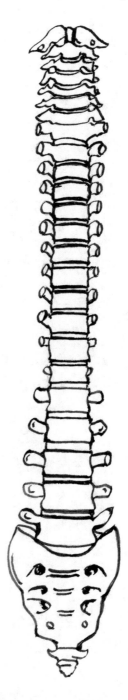

good abdominal muscle control, which in turn results in good trunk control and
greater balance. Damage here continues to impact bowel, bladder, and sexual
function.

Fig. 1.2 Spinal cord back
view; Mimi Smith

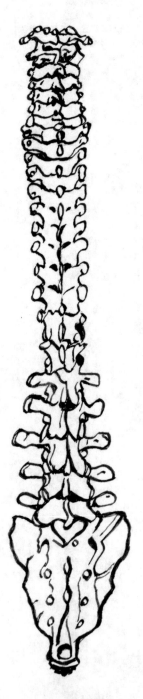

The lumbar and sacral spines are shorter in length than the thoracic spine. The lumbar spine runs from L1 to L5. Injuries in this level result in weakness and loss of motor control in the lower legs and can impact hip movements. Bowel, bladder, and

Fig. 1.3 Spinal cord side
view; Mimi Smith

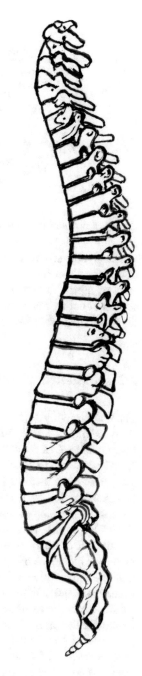

sexual function can also be affected in the upper lumbar spine. Because the nerves
that control these functions are located in the sacral spine, a lower level injury can
sometimes spare them.

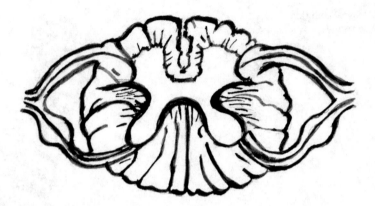

Fig. 1.4 Spinal cord cross section; Mimi Smith

Finally, the sacral spine runs from S1 to S5 and can result in some loss of function in the lower legs, as well as bowel bladder and sexual function. The lower the level of injury, the greater the probability that there will be more movement and control of bodily functions. The sacral spine is less flexible than the other regions of the spine and is fused to form the coccyx.

1.2 Statistical Considerations Around SCI

There are roughly 17,500 new cases a year. The average age of onset has gone up from 29 in the 1970s to 42 today. There is a strong gender discrepancy, with males making up 81% of the cases. Non-Hispanic whites have the greatest incidence with 63.3% compared to 21.7% of non-Hispanic blacks and 11.1% Hispanics since 2010. The cause remains most commonly vehicle accidents (38.4%), with falls (30.5%) and violence (13.5%) following behind. For level of injury, the greatest number consists of incomplete tetraplegia (45.8%), followed by incomplete paraplegia (20.9%), complete paraplegia (19.7%), and complete tetraplegia (13.2%) [1, 2].

Survival of cervical spine injuries has doubled since the 1970s, likely due to increased incidence of falls in the rising elderly population and due to advances in medical intervention with increased survival rates [3]. Mortality rates are high immediately after injury due to secondary conditions (traumatic brain injury) and cardiovascular or respiratory involvement [4]. In addition, the higher up the injury, the higher the rates of mortality, with a rate of 6.6% for C1–C3, 2.5% for C4–C5, and 1.5% for C6–C8 [5]. The second leading cause of death in individuals with SCI is septicemia (88.6%), usually associated with urinary tract infections (UTIs), pneumonia, or presence of pressure injury [6, 7].

1.3   Intervention: Medical

Acute and long-term complications can occur after spinal cord injury. These include problems with the lungs, heart, urinary tract, and bladder, spasticity, pain, pressure injury, heterotopic ossification, and osteoporosis.

1.3.1   Acute Intervention

While a spinal cord injury revolves around damage to the spine, there are many ancillary factors that must be examined. An entire examination of all systems needs to occur prior to arrival at the hospital and often even prior to transfer into the ambulance for transport. All systems can be impacted, including cardiovascular, respiratory, orthopedic, and neurological.

Each point of intervention is critical, from initial contact with the individual at the original location of the trauma, transport to the hospital, the emergency room, and so on. Research has indicated that 20% of those who have sustained spinal cord injury die prior to making it to the hospital [8]. For this reason it is essential proper intervention occurs from the moment the individual is assessed and intervention is provided. It cannot be stressed enough the importance of waiting for proper medical care to arrive after sustaining a spinal cord injury prior to moving the injured individual, unless absolutely necessary. Movement can lead to further damage to the spine and on occasion can be the primary factor that leads to total paralysis. Maintaining a stable spine is key to recovery.

While spinal trauma and other neurological impairment, including loss of consciousness, are of primary focus, initial contact by emergency personnel at the scene of the event must also examine other factors. Secondary factors come into play after the initial trauma. One primary need is oxygenation of the spinal cord. Impaired respiration leads to decreased oxygenation to the spinal cord which in turn leads to increased neuronal damage [3]. Hypoventilation, as well as aspiration, can occur from paralysis of the diaphragm or intercostal muscles. This can lead to respiratory and cardiac arrest, so it is essential that respiration is one of the first functions assessed. In addition, oxygenation must be assessed for cognitive function. Hypoxia can lead to brain damage, reinforcing the importance that oxygenation be assessed at all times. If it is found to be low, oxygen needs to be provided via a face mask or nasal cannula. Under extreme circumstances intubation should occur. This is when a tube is placed in the mouth and down the trachea to provide air directly to the lungs. Application of this however is risky since the spine must be stabilized. Stabilization is essential so as not to create further trauma to the spine or the body. Intubation requires hyperextension of the neck to ensure the tube can access the trachea. If it goes down the esophagus, it will not only provide much needed oxygen but will push air into the abdomen. Because intubation requires forcibly moving the cervical spine out of neutral and into extension, it occurs most commonly in the hospital setting upon arrival to the emergency department [9].

Another concern is neurogenic shock, which occurs when blood pools in the distal extremities. Due to the trauma to the system and the resultant shock, blood vessels don't properly circulate blood through the body. When this occurs, the individual has trouble stabilizing their heart rate, blood pressure, and temperature due to low blood flow. This can have deadly consequences. This is more common with those who sustain injury at T5 or above. The symptoms are fluctuations in heart rate, blood pressure, and temperature.

Stabilization is important prior to transporting the individual to the hospital. While research has shown that using a board with a cervical collar stabilized to the board with towel rolls by the head is best practice, it has also shown that there is a high incidence of pressure ulcer from prolonged contact with the board [9]. Peak pressures can be very high at both the sacral region of the spine and the occipital region of the skull [10]. While there are no real-time indicators, we know that prolonged pressure into tissues can cause damage to skin integrity (a topic explored at great length later on). This must also be a consideration during management of the acutely injured person with spinal cord injury prior to arrival at the hospital.

Generally, after sustaining a spinal cord injury, the individual is initially transferred to a hospital emergency room and then either to the neurological, trauma, or surgical intensive care unit (ICU) or the neurology department. From there, the person with SCI is most frequently transferred to a rehabilitation floor. There are multiple medical interventions that occur at various stages of the spinal cord injury. Timing of these interventions is dependent on the level of involvement, the severity of injury, and complications that can arise.

Surgery may be warranted, and timing of surgical intervention is dependent on several factors. Depending on the severity of injury and level of injury, there are occasions that emergency surgery will occur to repair vessels, bone, and soft tissue. At this time, emergent stabilization of the spine may also be necessary. On some occasions it is determined that waiting until the patient is more stable is better. Considerations are inflammation and fragility.

1.3.2 Assessment of Neurological Function

The initial assessment of neurological function occurs at the scene of the trauma. As incidence of death is very high at this moment, assessment at this time of all functions is critical. Loss of consciousness, complaints of pain, disorientation, and visible trauma are assessed. While it is important to identify locations of pain, the complaints do not always correlate to point of trauma. Not only can there be involvement of the spinal cord, but there can be internal organ damage as well, which can be both painful and life threatening. Furthermore, in the assessment of pain, it is important to be thorough as it has been found that in 15% of spinal cord injuries, there is another location of spinal trauma [8]. Upon this initial contact, the individual is questioned regarding their ability to move and their sensory response. However, it is not until arrival in the emergency room that true spinal involvement is assessed. It is here that diagnostic reflexes will occur to assess spinal levels.

Upon arrival to the hospital, a full body check of trauma occurs, including traumatic brain injury (TBI), organ involvement, and neurological impairment. Often times, radiological intervention is necessary to rule out further damage.

Neurological function in this population is assessed by checking sensory and reflex response. Various locations of the body are touched to determine whether the individual can feel tactile pressure. This is assessed along a dermatomal level that correlates to the spinal levels, looking at left and right sides. The transition from sensory awareness to inability to feel touch determines the level of sensory damage. The most distal level of response is identified as the diagnosed sensory level. In addition, motor responses and reflexes are assessed. The individual is asked to move various parts of their body. The most distal level of motor response is identified as the level of motor involvement. Like sensation, both left and right sides of the spinal cord are assessed. The most common reflexes assessed with this population are the anal reflex and the bulbocavernosus reflex. These are used to differentiate whether the injury is an upper motor neuron (UMN) or lower motor neuron (LMN) injury. UMN injuries generally result in increased spasticity, with sensory loss and bowel, bladder, and sexual dysfunction. LMN injuries result in flaccidity, sensory loss, and a loss of certain reflexes. If the reflex is intact, there is an UMN lesion and, if absent, a LMN lesion. Awareness of the type of lesion can help determine long-term bowel and bladder management [11].

In addition to the primary injury, there can be secondary traumas present. TBI is common with SCI when the nature of the injury is traumatic, as in the case of motor vehicle accidents, falls, assaults, and other high-force injuries. The rate of these can be as low as 40% [12]. This is an important consequence of SCI and can impact not only the individual's ability to learn new skills but also their behavior and willingness to participate. For this reason, often times neuropsychological testing will occur once the patient is stable or on the rehabilitation unit.

1.3.3 Orthopedic Repair or Stabilization of the Spine

It has been determined that for cervical spine injuries, spinal stabilization needs to occur within 24 hours. Early surgical decompression can result in improved neurological outcome over time [13, 14]. Research has also found that the window for surgery for thoracic spine injuries is also 24 hours. This amount of time has been found to decrease ICU stay and the need for ventilator assistance [15].

1.3.4   Exploratory Surgery for Soft Tissue Damage

After a traumatic SCI, there is often damage to soft tissues. Whether the traumatic event is forceful (i.e., a motor vehicle accident) or the result of external trauma (i.e., a gunshot wound), tissues can tear both externally and internally.

After trauma, several complications can occur, including rib fractures and organ contusions, lacerations, or ruptures. When there is respiratory trauma, sometimes a thoracostomy is required (chest tube placement to drain fluid and blood). Ruptures to organs require emergent removal or repair, whereas contusions and lacerations will often require vigilant observation to assess changes over time. These changes can happen quickly, so constant monitoring is essential [16].

If the SCI is a result of gunshot wound (GSW), intervention is dependent on the level of injury and the nature of the trauma. GSW to the cervical spine run the risk of impacting the airway and the major arteries traveling in the neck. The thoracic spine is most commonly impacted by GSW [17]. Imaging is used to determine location of bullet or bullet fragments. There are often incidences when the bullet and fragments are not surgically removed. This occurs when removal will result in greater trauma than if they are left in place.

1.3.5   Respiratory Considerations

Respiratory complications lead to the highest incidence of mortality in spinal cord injury [18]. Eighty percent of deaths of those with cervical spine injuries are due to respiratory dysfunction, with pneumonia causing 50% of them [16]. The higher the level of injury and increased time since injury results in greater decrease in lung volume [19]. Respiratory complications in this population increase within the first 3–5 days [16]. This often can result in a higher risk of pneumonia due to paralysis of respiratory muscles and a decreased cough reflex [20].

External ventilation can be warranted both after initial injury and over time. Depending on the level of injury or neurologic impairment, respiratory muscles may be affected. The diaphragm is essential for breathing. Innervation of the diaphragm occurs around C4. Therefore, an individual with a complete SCI at the level of C6 would likely have impairment of some muscles responsible for inspiration and expiration. However, the diaphragm would be spared. This individual would be able to breathe without external mechanical ventilator assistance. However, an individual with a complete lesion at C2 would have some form of paralysis of the diaphragm and would therefore require mechanical ventilation [21].

Another long-term consideration is tracheal scarring and lacerations, which can occur from intubation and surgical spine stabilization. The scar tissue can affect fluidity of movement of these tissues and result in long-term damage.

1.3.6 Acute Use of Steroids and Cold

Steroids and cold are often used to decrease inflammation and encourage vascularization. Immediately after the initial trauma, there is damage to tissues. Tissue damage however continues to occur due to hypoxia and toxicity. When trauma occurs, the body releases proteins and free radicals which result in inflammation and tissue destruction. Cell death advances over time. It begins within minutes and upward of weeks as metabolic changes lead from one event to another. For this reason, function isn't always clear immediately after the initial trauma, because cells that initially survived the injury can ultimately die, leading to permanent damage.

However, slowing down the inflammation and hypoxia can decrease the effect of damage. Therefore, because hypoxia and ischemia worsen the damage to the nervous system, use of steroids and cold becomes an important part of treatment both initially and over time. Oftentimes, emergency service vehicles are equipped with cold blankets to cover the trauma patient during transport to the emergency department.

1.4 Medical Consequences of SCI

There are multiple medical consequences that occur as a result of SCI. These can be acute and chronic and can have severe ramifications in long-term survival. In this section, the most common consequences and symptoms will be explored, in no order of specificity or priority.

1.4.1 Pressure Injuries

A pressure injury is a localized injury to the skin and/or underlying tissue due to either pressure or a combination of pressure and shear. They usually occur over a bony prominence and areas that sustain greater pressure, including the "butt bones" (ischial tuberosities), the "tail bone" (sacrum and coccyx), the "hip bones" (trochanters), the "shoulder blades" (scapula), the heels and ankles, and the back of the head. They occur due to the inability to sense pressure. Nerve endings send information through the nervous system to the brain when there is something noxious to the system, like increased or prolonged pressure. The brain then reacts and sends information to the muscles to move the body. However, with spinal cord injury, these pathways of information are often damaged. The result is this information does not get transmitted to the brain and in turn the brain cannot react. The individual remains in the same position for a prolonged time cutting off blood flow to the area.

Blood provides nutrients and oxygen throughout the body. When blood flow stops, tissues are deprived of nutrients and oxygen. This results in localized tissue death with inflammation to the surrounding areas. Even once the pressure is removed, not only has the tissue already died, but the inflammation interferes in resumption of healthy blood flowing into the area. This impacts length of time for healing to occur.

Pressure injuries are the second most frequent complication in individuals with spinal cord injury [7]. Approximately 15–33% of people with spinal cord injury will have an incidence of skin impairment at some point in their lives, with a recurrence rate of up to 60%.

The National Pressure Ulcer Advisory Panel (NPUAP) changed its name to the National Pressure Injury Advisory Panel (NPIAP) and its terminology from pressure ulcer to pressure injury on April 16, 2016 [22]. An ulcer by definition is an open wound. However, damage to tissue from pressure doesn't always include an open wound. Pressure occurs from the inside out so the onset of development of the injury in its nature is not necessarily a wound. Therefore, to provide greater guidelines for intervention, the terminology was changed to address the impairment to skin integrity that occurs without the presence of an open wound. However, common vernacular remains pressure ulcer among many in this population.

The six different stages of pressure ulcer (injury) identified in the NPIAP Guidelines are stage 1, stage 2, stage 3, stage 4, unstageable, and deep tissue pressure injury. A stage 1 pressure injury is a non-blanchable erythema of intact skin. The skin pigmentation is darker and does not blanch (lighten) when pressure is applied to it. There may also be changes in temperature or firmness prior to change in color (Fig. 1.5). A stage 2 pressure injury is classified as a partial-thickness skin loss with exposed dermis. The wound bed is usually pink or red and can present as a ruptured blister (Fig. 1.6). A stage 3 injury consists of full-thickness skin loss. Fat is visible, with granulation and rolled wound edges present. Undermining and tunneling can occur. Tunneling is when the wound travels deep into tissues under the surface. Tunneling needs to be measured to determine true stage of injury. Though these wounds are deeper, they do not go deeper than the overlying skin layers (Fig. 1.7). That occurs with stage 4 injuries, which are full-thickness skin and tissue injuries. Tissue loss here results in exposure of the fascia, muscle, tendon, ligament, cartilage, and bone. Again, rolled skin edges, undermining, and tunneling can occur (Fig. 1.8). The following two categories refer to injuries that cannot be staged as it is unclear what is occurring. The first, unstageable pressure injury, refers to skin loss that is covered with slough or eschar. It is not until this covering is removed that we can see what underneath is in regard to staging the injury (Fig. 1.9). Finally, a deep tissue pressure injury is one that does not blanche when touched and that presents as red, maroon, or purple in color. This indicates that under the surface there is a deep wound present. Unlike stage 1 where this is more superficial, this injury is much deeper, and it is not until it opens up that we can classify its stage.

In addition to direct pressure, there are other mechanical processes that occur that can result in pressure injuries, including shear, friction, and force. Shear forces are forces that occur parallel to the skin. Friction is the sliding of two forces with respect to each other. Loaded forces result in strain and stress, creating deformation of the tissues. All factors can directly result in pressure injuries [23]. Newer research

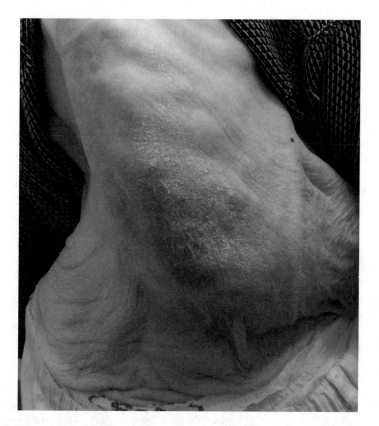

Fig. 1.5 Stage 1 pressure injury

identifies that the impact from loaded forces can cause the greatest damage due to the extent of deformation.

There are external and internal causes of pressure injury. External causes are pressure, shear, friction, and force. Internal causes are loss of muscle mass, decreased circulation, moisture from sweating and incontinence, weight gain or loss, spasticity, aging, and history of previous breakdown. Factors such as the skin becoming weaker and thinner through illness or aging, or skin becoming macerated through moisture and incontinence, affect the superficial layers of the skin and make them more likely to tear. Muscle wasting and weight loss decrease the amount of mass between the bony prominence and the skin surface increasing the potential of forces affecting the tissues. A previous history of skin injury results in scar tissue. Scar tissue is unlike healthy skin in that it binds differently, so when shear, force, and pressure occur, there is tearing to the scar tissue. Spasticity is an interesting concept. Spasticity, which will be discussed further in this chapter, is an over-firing of nerves into the muscle resulting in the muscle contracting at a high rate. Increased spasticity can result in the increase of muscle mass, which protects the skin. However, it can also result in shear, which damages the skin.

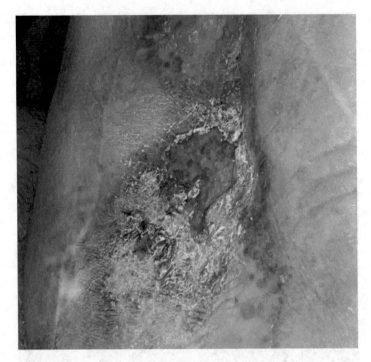

Fig. 1.6 Stage 2 pressure injury

Time since onset of spinal cord injury also plays a large role. Over time the risk for development of injury increases. It's been found that 2 years post injury, the incidence can be as high as 31% at the ischium, 26% at the trochanters, and 18% at the sacrum [24].

Pressure injuries are common but not guaranteed. Though several factors, as identified above, play a role, changing one's position frequently can dramatically decrease the onset of ulcer. The common belief is positional change every 30–60 minutes for 3–5 minutes at a time which will significantly decrease the potential for development of pressure injury.

There are many ways to change one's position, dependent on the level of spinal cord injury and the complex rehabilitation technology wheelchair being used. When seated in a power wheelchair that has power seat functions, the best way to relieve pressure is to tilt the entire seat back 45 degrees and recline the backrest 120 degrees. When seated in a manual wheelchair, the best way to relieve pressure is to either bend forward onto one's lap or lean to the side, alternating between the left and right. These positions need to be sustained for 3–5 minutes to encourage full reperfusion of blood into the areas bearing weight. They should also occur every 30–60 minutes.

Treatment for these injuries can range from use of medications and wound dressings to surgery. Surgical interventions include debridement and flap surgery. Debridement is a cleaning of the wound by removal of the dead tissue. This can

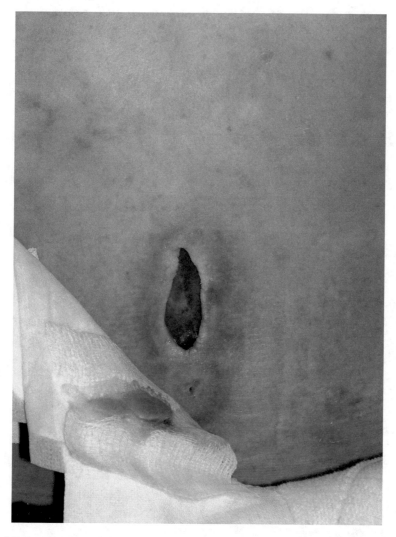

Fig. 1.7 Stage 3 pressure injury

often result in a larger wound as the dead tissue is removed, but what is left is healthy tissue. When the wound is deeper and is unable to heal after debridement, reconstructive surgery is often necessary. Known as a "flap" surgery, the skin is placed over the wound to provide blood flow to the wound area. The "flap" of the muscle and tissue is placed over the wound, usually still partially attached, to provide a source of blood and nutrients to travel to the wound to encourage healing. The injuries that usually require these surgical interventions are stage 3 and 4 as these wounds are often too deep to heal on their own [25].

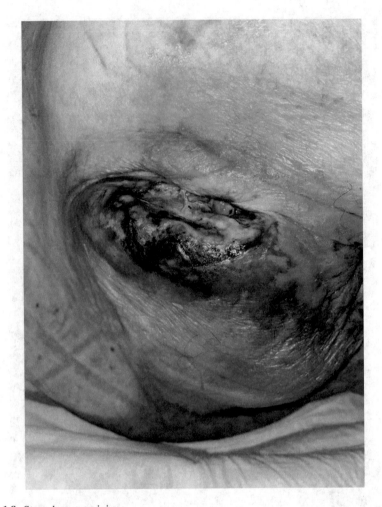

Fig. 1.8 Stage 4 pressure injury

1.4.2 Pain

Pain is another common symptom experienced after sustaining a spinal cord injury
[26, 27]. The rates can be as low as 11% and as high as 94% [28]. For most persons
with SCI, the development of pain is found to increase over time [29].

Chronic pain is common with spinal cord injury, lasting months to years. There
are several pain types affecting several different parts of the body. This pain can
usually be managed to a point that it does not interfere in function, but in order to
determine the root cause, tests are necessary. The most frequently experienced types
of pain in SCI are neuropathic pain, visceral pain, upper limb pain, and back pain.
Back pain can be either neuropathic or musculoskeletal [30].

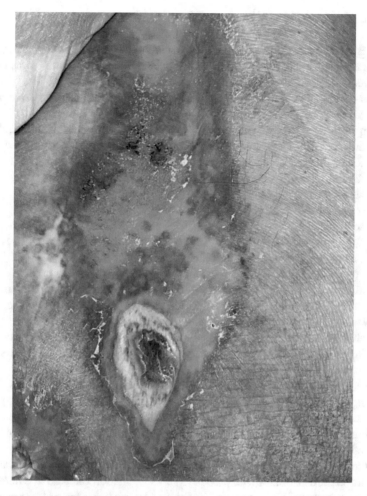

Fig. 1.9 Unstageable pressure injury

Upper limb pain is most frequently correlated with wheelchair design and configuration, as well as functional task technique. Overuse comes most frequently from wheelchair propulsion. It can also come from transfers and functional activities. Frequent use of the muscles in the upper extremities leads to inflammation which leads to pain. The result is decreased ability to function. This pain can be located in the shoulders, elbows, wrists, and hands [26, 31]. Among persons with SCI, research has found pain in the hand and wrist to occur between 15% and 48% of the time, in the elbow between 22% and 45% as well as aspiration, and in the shoulder between 30% and 60% as well as aspiration [32]. While this range is extensive, it identifies that at least a quarter of the population of persons with SCI will develop elbow pain and a third shoulder pain. This is a large number and must be addressed for proper intervention with persons with SCI. Sie et al. [33] found that pain that impacts daily function is present in 59% of the persons with tetraplegia and 41% of the persons with paraplegia.

As it relates to mobility, pain has been found to be both caused by and relieved by wheelchair use. For many with chronic upper extremity pain, often transitioning to powered mobility is essential. This is supported in the literature, identifying significant decrease in complaints of pain and mobility with the use of powered mobility [34].

Pain is experienced when information is sent up and down the nerves to and from the brain and various locations of the body. With neuropathic pain, due to damage to the nerves from the spinal cord injury, these signals do not travel as they once did. The body has difficulty understanding these signals resulting in pain being experienced below the level of injury. This pain can be burning, tingling, or stabbing. This pain is often hard to treat as it is neurological in nature.

Musculoskeletal pain originates from the muscles, joints, and bones. It can be postural, positional, repetitive, or mechanical. Postural and positional causes are often a result of poor positioning in the wheelchair or the bed. When poorly supported, these complaints will increase. It is common for wheelchair users to develop complaints of lower back pain due to lack of support to the trunk. Research has shown that lumbar support combined with ten degrees of an open seat to back angle can take pressure off the lower back when seated. By providing proper seating, the experience of musculoskeletal pain can decrease. Musculoskeletal pain can also occur in patients who have undergone spinal surgery due to trauma to the tissues as well as the strain on the muscles above and below the surgery.

Spasticity can create mechanical pain, with over-firing of the nervous system resulting in repetitive muscle contractions. Spasticity will be discussed in greater detail below, but the over-firing of muscles creates cramping and fatigue, which can lead to intense pain. This is usually treated with weight-bearing activities and anti-spasmodic pharmaceuticals.

Visceral pain is often referred pain. When there is damage to the spinal cord, nerve information cannot travel properly. This information can lead to alteration in sensation viscerally. It is important to make sure however that there is nothing medically going on and if the person with SCI is experiencing visceral pain, they should contact their physician. The person with SCI may not know this is visceral pain. But pain that is located in the flank or the trunk should be investigated by a physician as it can often be associated with urological symptoms.

There are various treatments for pain, including physical, psychological, and pharmaceutical. It is important to discuss with a physician the type of pain the person with SCI is experiencing. Being specific as to time of day, onset and triggers will aid the physician in determining the best intervention.

Physical interventions can be broken down into treatment and positioning. Treatments include physical and occupational therapy and modalities. Physical and occupational therapists can provide manual therapy, including massage. Massage can aid in releasing muscles and fascia, which in turn can decrease muscle tightness and complaints of pain. Sometimes they combine this with modalities such as electrical stimulation. Electrical stimulation enters the body through pads adhered to the skin. It creates an electrical current which can interrupt the abnormal nerve signals causing pain. Acupuncture can be used as well to treat pain and should only be administered by a certified and trained acupuncturist. Corticosteroid injections can also be beneficial in decreasing inflammation in a localized area. Orthotics can be used to stabilize an area and decrease inflammation from positioning. For example, a resting hand splint can stabilize the wrist in neutral to decrease pressure along the carpal tunnel from increased flexion or extension and in turn decrease complaints of pain.

Medications are often used as well, ranging from muscle relaxants to pain meds depending on the severity and location. It is important to work with a physiatrist or pain management physician with good understanding of SCI when addressing medication management.

1.4.3   Spasticity Management

Spasticity affects 70% of the persons with SCI [35]. Spasticity is an involuntary contraction of muscles. It occurs when information cannot be properly sent along the nervous system. Under normal circumstances, when stimuli presents itself (either noxious or simple sensory input), this information travels from the sensory nerves at the point of the stimulus up the spinal cord to the brain. The brain interprets this data and sends a response down the spinal column for the motor nerves to respond. Reflexive responses occur more immediately. When the spinal cord is damaged, the information traveling up the spinal column cannot travel past the point of damage. It cannot make it to the brain for a response. Rather, it travels up the spine, hits the point of damage, and reflexively travels back down.

Spasticity can be triggered by simple sensory stimuli or movement. Spasticity is also a valuable tool in the determination that there is something amiss medically. Certain medical symptoms can trigger spasm, including a pressure injury, UTI, or fracture. For this reason, if a new onset or worsening of spasticity develops, it is essential to pursue medical intervention.

When spasticity occurs, muscles tighten with repeated contractions. This can occur anywhere in the body, predominantly in the limbs, back, and neck. However, spasticity can also occur in the trunk and abdomen. The presentation can be muscles contracting into extension with the legs, trunk, and arms straightening or flexion with the joints bending inward. Hands can close into a fist or clasped position. Repeated contractions can present as a muscle spasm and clonus.

Along with the physical symptoms, sensory symptoms develop as well. This includes sensations of heat and intense pain. When spasm occurs in the chest, difficulty of breathing can occur. Spasticity can be so intense that it can cause someone to slide out of their wheelchair. This creates shear at the surface of the body contacting the wheelchair and can negatively impact skin integrity. Repetitive spasticity causes constant contracture around a joint and can ultimately result in loss of range of motion.

Along with the negative consequences, there are benefits to spasticity. Spasticity causes multiple muscle contractions. This can result in constant increased muscle bulk, weight shift, and pressure relief. Spasticity can also aid in activities of daily living. Spasticity can result in hand closure around objects or can assist in body movements when performing certain activities such as transfers.

Spasticity management becomes essential for the SCI population [36]. Spasticity can negatively impact quality of life, causing pain and decreased function. For this reason, there are several interventions that exist. Interventions are mechanical, pharmacological, and surgical. Weight bearing has been shown to decrease onset of spasm and decrease spasm at time of onset. Daily range of motion can also decrease onset by maintaining flexibility. There are also positions that can aid in decreasing onset. When seated, increased hip and knee flexion can decrease onset of extension. Additionally, when pressure is applied into the ball of the foot, spasms can be triggered. Providing support to the entire bottom of the foot decreases localized pressure into the ball and in turn decreases onset of triggering spasm. Sometimes braces are used for control. These are most effective distally at the wrist and hand, ankle, and foot [37].

There are two forms of pharmacological intervention: oral meds and muscle injections or nerve blocks. Oral meds can be effective, but they have side effects that can be intense. Side effects include fatigue, dry mouth and increased thirst, dizziness, nausea, and even sometimes lowering of blood pressure. Many individuals with spinal cord injury are already experiencing these symptoms, so increasing them is not a desired outcome.

A common surgical intervention is implantation of an intrathecal device, also known as a baclofen pump [37]. A small battery-powered device is implanted into the abdominal wall with a tube (catheter) weaving into the spinal canal. A dose of baclofen, predetermined by a physician, is slowly released into the spine. Unlike oral medications, the number of side effects dramatically decreases since it is not being released into the bloodstream. So, the effects of fatigue and increased thirst are not present. A consideration of the pump is its life span. The pump needs to be replaced every 5–7 years, requiring additional future surgeries to remove and replace the device. There are other risks with this too, including the risk of over- or underdosing. Any disruption in the flow of baclofen into the nervous system can cause a chain reaction, resulting in the potential for stroke, heart attack, and ultimately death. There is an alarm set that ensures regular refill of the baclofen into the pump. However, there is the potential for alarm failure or catheter blockage. So, it is very important to be in contact with your physician. If the person with SCI notices changes in spasticity, including headaches, body aches, sweating, or increased spasticity, contact a physician immediately as this can be a life-threatening event.

1.4.4 Bladder and Bowel Function

After spinal cord injury, bowel and bladder functions are usually affected. Both functions are essential for health and function. Likewise, damage to both systems can affect every aspect of the individual, including physical health and mental well-being. Level of injury and completeness of injury can determine if the bowel and bladder are impacted.

Urination is a multiple-step process. The kidneys create urine, urine travels down the ureters to the bladder, and urine empties out of the bladder through a sphincter and then travels down the urethra. Some of these functions are autonomic. They are controlled by the autonomic nervous system and are not altered due to damage to the spinal cord. However, the bladder and sphincter are muscles, controlled by the nervous system. So, damage to the spinal cord affects how these muscles react. These muscles can become flaccid or spastic.

When the bladder is flaccid, the reflexes are slowed down or absent. The bladder can become extended and back up into the ureters and the kidneys, and urine may leak out. Prolonged stretching can cause long-term damage to the tone of the bladder. When the bladder is spastic, as urine fills the bladder, a reflex is triggered to empty the bladder. However, this can occur at any time and sometimes doesn't occur at all. This can be very dangerous, resulting in autonomic dysreflexia, which will be discussed later. The sphincter needs to relax to let urine out of the bladder into the urethra. If it doesn't relax, urine can back up in the bladder and in turn into the kidneys. If constantly relaxed, urine will leak out into the urethra.

There are different interventions dependent on the type of dysfunction. Catheterization is a common intervention. There are three common techniques: external condom catheter, indwelling catheter, and intermittent catheterization. The external condom catheter consists of a condom secured to the penis with a tube that empties out into a bag. An indwelling catheter is a catheter that is placed inside the urethra up into the bladder. It empties into a bag at the other end of the catheter. The most common form of catheterization is intermittent catheterization. Intermittent catheterization occurs roughly every 4 hours to ensure full release of urine from the bladder. A common long-term solution is a suprapubic catheter. A suprapubic catheter is a tube that is inserted directly into the bladder through a hole in the abdomen. Urine is directly drained out of this tube. For persons with impaired hand function (tetraplegia) or with chronic UTI, this can be an effective alternative. A conversation with your physiatrist and urologist can help you determine which intervention will best meet your needs.

Consequences around incontinence can be serious. UTI are common and can be hard to treat. Hydration and catherization in a sterile environment can keep a urinary system healthy. But, sometimes, infections of varying intensity develop. Treatment includes the use of oral antibiotics. However, infections can become unresponsive to antibiotics. The more frequent the UTI, the less effective the antibiotics can become, having one to use different antibiotics over time. On occasion, intravenous antibiotics are the best treatment option. The infection can become so severe it leads to infection and damage to the kidneys. This can lead to sepsis and under worst circumstances death. For this reason, it is important to focus on bladder management early for long-term health.

UTI can also lead to autonomic dysreflexia, which will be discussed later. This is dangerous and can cause various cardiovascular events and even death. For this reason, it is essential to be on top of one's bladder regimen.

A bowel movement occurs when waste is passed out of your colon, through your bowel and ultimately out of the body via the anus. When someone has experienced a spinal cord injury, this can be impacted. Spasticity and low tone affect this process differently resulting in either constipation and retention of stool (flaccidity) or in incontinence (spasticity).

Constipation is a common symptom among persons with spinal cord injury due to immobility and medication side effects. Immobility directly affects motility, interfering in the digestion process. Additionally, a common side effect of medication use is constipation.

A bowel program is an effective way to manage bowel incontinence and decrease the risk of constipation or bowel accidents. A bowel program consists of a coordinated intervention of medications and stimulation, as well as proper hydration and dietary intake. A proper diet, high in fiber and hydration, can help encourage regular elimination. In addition, use of laxatives and other stimulants can facilitate a bowel movement. However, this alone does not guarantee regular timing of a bowel routine. Sometimes techniques are required. The primary techniques are digital stimulation, digital removal, and insertion of enemas.

Digital stimulation consists of using a fingertip performing small rotational movements around the anus. These occur for 20 seconds at a time and should be performed every 5–10 minutes until the bowel movement is completed. Digital removal consists of using your finger to actively remove stool from the rectum. Sometimes one of these techniques will be adequate to complete your bowel routine, but sometimes you may need to use more than just one. This process can take time to perform. For many with SCI, their morning routine takes an excessive amount of time.

On occasion there are surgical techniques that need to be pursued if the above techniques are not effective. A colostomy can allow for independent management of bowel due to easier access. This is a surgical procedure where a portion of the colon is diverted to an opening in the abdomen, with stool emptying into a bag. Like a suprapubic catheter, this can more easily be accessed due to proximity. However, there can also be complications, which is why it is often considered as the technique of last resort by many. For persons with pressure injury a colostomy can remove feces from open infected tissue, encouraging a drier cleaner area and promote healing. Communicating with your physiatrist regarding techniques and options is very important.

Like bladder incontinence, bowel incontinence can lead to several secondary symptoms and complications. These include gas, bloating, heartburn, hemorrhoids, nausea, and pain, with more dangerous complications such as autonomic dysreflexia, stomach paralysis, and ulcers. Managing your bowel regimen is therefore extremely important and can lead to severe complications.

Loss of bowel and bladder function can lead to decreased community engagement due to fear of having an accident when out in the community. Many persons with SCI identify shame and embarrassment over leakage. This makes development of a bowel and bladder program essential for life satisfaction.

1.4.5 Sexual Health

There are several considerations around the concept of sexual health and sexuality. The cognitive emotional component plays a very large role here as there is often an alteration in personal identity post spinal cord injury. This component will be explored in greater detail in Chap. 3. The focus in this section will be on the physical manifestations. In addition, fertility and conception will be examined.

After a spinal cord injury, sexual function is affected. The extent of the impact is determined by the level of injury or completeness of injury. This is due to the effect on sensory and motor nerves. Arousal and the physical act of engaging in intercourse require a combination of sensory and motor function.

For men, the primary impact is on erectile dysfunction, ejaculation, and fertility and, for women, complaints of pain or orgasm. A large component of arousal, in men and women, is psychogenic. For men, reflexive arousal is also a very important component to the process.

Psychogenic arousal occurs when sexual thoughts, sights, sounds, and smells turn a person on. Cognitive thought and psychological experience create physiological responses such as increased heart rate and blood pressure, which in turn can lead to an erection in men or increased vaginal lubrication in women. With spinal cord injury, some of the responses to such thoughts are altered. It becomes important to explore with your body to determine how to recreate this sense of arousal. Touch can be used effectively, but with higher levels of injury and incomplete injuries, psychogenic arousal can be more problematic. Reflex arousal in men occurs around S2–S4 and is possible with a spinal cord injury above T10.

As stated above, location and completeness result in different reactions. To review, upper motor neurons are located in the spinal cord and brain. Lower motor neurons are located in the spinal cord and brain stem. Lower motor neurons connect the upper motor neurons and skeletal muscles. A complete upper motor neuron injury will usually result with no psychogenic erection for men, but a reflex erection. However, an incomplete upper motor neuron injury could have both present, whereas a complete lower motor neuron injury in the sacral spine usually results in psychogenic erection but no reflex erection [38].

For the treatment of lack of erection, there are several interventions. There are oral pharmacological options, dermatological pharmacological interventions, intravenous options, use of external devices, and, in very limited situations, prosthetics. Advances in pharmacology have provided men with spinal cord injury several different medications to choose from, usually resulting in an effective response with one. The medications can prolong the erection or increase the frequency of it. External devices, such as rings, can be used to maintain increased blood flow into the penis after erection is achieved to prolong its effect. These options are all generally effective. On very rare circumstances, there is the need for prosthetics. These are generally more necessary when there is a reconstructive issue or damage to the tissue.

Ejaculation and orgasm require a synchronized interaction between the sympathetic, parasympathetic, and somatic sensory systems. When damage occurs to the spinal cord, this movement pattern is often not in harmony. Depending on the level or completeness of the injury, there can be orgasm, but no ejaculation, ejaculation without orgasm, or minimal effect of either. The more incomplete the injury, the greater the likelihood that both will occur.

Infertility in men is a result of time. Shortly after injury, sperm maintains a high level of motility and viability. However, over time this diminishes, and sperm loses its strength and effectiveness [39]. Some causes are frequent UTI, retrograde ejaculation, problems with temperature regulation, and medications. If the long-term goal is to have a child, sperm banking is often recommended.

There is less research regarding women. However, this has changed over time, with increased focus on how damage to the nervous system affects women's ability to experience sexual pleasure and how spinal cord injury impacts women's fertility. Women experience psychogenic arousal as well as a form of reflex arousal. For women, there are fewer physiological interruptions, with the primary component of sexual health affected being lubrication. The generation of natural lubricant occurs when nerve signals are sent to the genital area. With a spinal cord injury, these nerves can become damaged resulting in the decreased generation of lubrication. However, there are pharmacological options to manage this.

Arousal for women is usually unchanged. However, loss of sensation and motor control can impact a woman's ability to experience pleasure. Sensory changes impact the ability to sense internal and tactile stimulation, while the lack of motor control can affect muscle contractions. Exploring alternative positions provides opportunities to achieve sexual pleasure. To achieve this there are not only tools available, but also furniture options to facilitate maintaining a specific position (i.e., IntimateRider).

After sustaining a spinal cord injury, menstruation can stop for a short period of time. When this occurs, fertility is affected. However, once one's period returns, the ability to become pregnant returns. Becoming pregnant is generally not a problem for women with spinal cord injury. However, sustaining a pregnancy can be more challenging. The lack of muscle tone below the level of injury, spasticity, and secondary complications such as autonomic dysreflexia or orthostatic hypotension can all affect a woman's ability to carry a child to term.

For both men and women, there are certain considerations. Bowel and bladder functions are of concern, with apprehension of emptying during sexual activities. It is recommended that emptying occurs prior to any sexual activity to decrease the risk of this. There are deeper, more personal concerns as well, which will be explored in greater detail in Chap. 3. However, they are important to mention here. After a spinal cord injury, the individual experiences an altered sense of self. This not only impacts the sense of one's body in space or ones perceived body functions, but it also impacts ones perceived sense of physical and sexual attraction. This needs to be explored as loneliness is a factor of recovery.

1.4.6   Respiratory Complications

Respiration is vital to all aspects of function. The process of respiration consists of two stages: inhalation and exhalation. Inhalation is an active process, while exhalation is a passive one. In order to inhale, the muscles need to activate to affect the diaphragm, the chest, the neck, and the abdomen. These muscles require nerve function to be elicited. When inhaling, the diaphragm drops, the intercostal muscles and neck muscles expand the muscles of the chest to allow the lungs to fill, and the abdomen expands to allow for taking a deep breath and coughing as needed. All four muscle groups work in conjunction to ensure effective inhalation.

Depending on the level of injury, respiratory function can be affected. An injury above T12 will affect respiration, since T1 to T12 is where control of the abdominal and intercostal muscles is located. When these muscles are not enervated, the ability to expand the abdomen and chest impacts the ability to fully inhale. Diaphragm control is situated around C3 to C5, so damage above this area of the spine results in the inability to inhale, often requiring external assistance to breath. Under these circumstances, the patient requires the use of a ventilator. However, long-term need of a ventilator is usually only necessary with complete injuries above C3. Usually below this level the patient can be weaned off the ventilator either full time or part time, requiring use at night only.

Respiratory complications can occur after spinal cord injury, regardless of the level of injury or completeness. Possible complications include atelectasis, pulmonary embolism (PE), and pneumonia. Atelectasis is when the lung collapses and cannot fill up with air. Though not as common as the others, it can happen and requires emergent intervention to ensure full lung inflation. Pulmonary embolism occurs when a blood clot blocks the blood vessels leading to the lungs. Persons with SCI are at high risk for PE due to immobility. Lack of muscle contractions to pump blood through the body and metabolic changes can result in the blood clotting. Treatment includes medications that thin the blood and implantation of a greenfield filter. This is a procedure where a mesh filter is surgically placed through the groin into the inferior vena cava. The filter holes are large enough to allow for blood to easily move through but small enough to catch clots and prevent them from traveling up into the lungs.

Pneumonia is the most common respiratory complication among persons with higher level SCI. It is also the leading cause of death among persons with cervical SCI. It is important to be aware of the symptoms of pneumonia due to the serious risk of illness and mortality. Symptoms include shortness of breath, congestion, fever, cough, and pallor.

Treatments for respiratory complications include chest physical therapy and a cough assist machine. Both use a form of percussion to stimulate the lungs and cause phlegm to be released from the tissue. Coughing aides in the removal of congestion and decreases the incidence of pneumonia. Other interventions include maintaining a healthy weight, hydration, exercise, and a good diet. Another key intervention is posture and positioning. It is important to maintain an open chest cavity to encourage air to freely move in and out of the lungs. This can occur with a proper seating system in one's wheelchair. Power seat functions on a power wheelchair may allow for dynamic positional change to ensure a postural tolerance. Seating and positioning will be explored more fully later in this book.

1.4.7 Autonomic Dysreflexia

Autonomic dysreflexia (AD) is a very dangerous condition. It usually affects individuals with a spinal cord injury above T5 or T6, though it has been found in persons with a T7 or T8 injury. When a noxious stimulus occurs, usually something painful, this information is sent to the spinal cord via nerve impulses and then up the spine to the brain to respond. However, when someone has a spinal cord injury and they experience stimuli below their level of injury, the information travels along the spine until the point of injury and is blocked. The information cannot reach the brain and the body cannot respond normally. A reflex is triggered that directly affects the sympathetic portion of the autonomic nervous system, causing a narrowing of blood vessels and a rise in blood pressure. For those with no damage to their autonomic nervous system, when this occurs, nerve receptors in the heart trigger the brain to slow down the heart rate and relax the blood vessels. However, for a person with a spinal cord injury above T5 or T6, this does not occur, and blood pressure cannot be regulated. This becomes an extremely dangerous situation and can lead to heart attack, seizure, and stroke and can result in death [40].

Possible causes of this can be a pressure injury, a UTI, a blocked or tangled catheter, a full bladder or bowel, a broken bone, or an ingrown toenail. There is also a higher risk during menstruation and sexual activity. Another consideration is body art, including piercing and tattooing. Anything that causes pressure into tissues that are in excess of their tolerance can cause AD.

AD symptoms run the range of increased sweating above level of injury, sweating on half of the body or face, slowed heart rate, clammy skin below level of injury, goosebumps, chills, flushed skin, or pounding headache. When these symptoms occur, the person with SCI should check their blood pressure. It is important to have a good baseline knowledge of one's blood pressure to better monitor health and incidence of dysreflexia. While determining the cause of AD, it is important to consistently check blood pressure until symptoms subside. After the initial blood pressure check, the person with SCI should begin exploring possible causes of AD. Loosen tight clothing, check to see if the bladder is full or if the catheter is kinked, check the skin along the seated surface for redness or breakdown, make sure the bowel is not full, and check for bruising to see if a bone has been broken. Due to sensory loss from the spinal cord injury, it is possible to sustain a significant injury, like a fracture, and not feel it.

1.4.8 Orthostatic Hypotension

Orthostatic hypotension (OH) is a decrease in blood pressure within 3 minutes of standing. The sympathetic and parasympathetic nervous systems are responsible for the management of blood pressure. The parasympathetic system lowers blood rate, while the sympathetic system increases it. When the sympathetic system is triggered, there is an increase in peripheral vascular flow and in turn blood pressure. The vascular system prevents pooling of blood and maintains healthy blood pressure. However, when there is damage to this system, there is damage to the spinal cardiovascular pathways, resulting in the over-stimulation of the sympathetic system. Damage to the spine not only interferes with normal processing of motor and sensory functions, it also interferes in cardiovascular processing that happens in the thoracic spine. Because this is not functioning well, orthostatic hypotension occurs. In addition, the lack of skeletal muscle in the lower extremities impacts the ability to pump out pooling fluid. Another factor is impaired baroreceptors. Baroreceptors modulate the sympathetic and parasympathetic systems reflexively to maintain blood pressure. Baroreceptor function has found to be defective in a person with SCI above T3 [41]. For this reason, persons with SCI often have a baseline blood pressure that is lower [42].

When the person with SCI moves from supine to sitting, they can develop symptoms of dizziness, lightheadedness, and even syncopal events due to drops in heart rate and blood pressure. OH has been found present in 74% of the persons with SCI, with symptoms of lightheadedness and dizziness in 59% of persons with SCI [43]. Treatment can include wearing compression garments or an abdominal binder.

The experience of OH is scary. Persons with SCI are already in a state of loss of control of their body due to all the factors discussed in this section. It is imperative that persons with SCI are giving knowledge on OH and supported both physically and emotionally through the process. Education on the causes and symptoms can decrease the severity of the outcome.

1.4.9 Bone Health

The two primary considerations for bone health among this population are osteoporosis and heterotopic ossification. They are both two very different processes that occur and can impact function and quality of life differently.

Osteoporosis is a loss of bone density. It occurs rapidly in the first 12–18 months and then continues over time [44]. Factors leading to onset of osteoporosis are diet, medications, and weight bearing. For persons with SCI, the loss of the ability to walk results in decreased weight bearing into bones and joints and leads to the destruction of bone density. It is usually assessed using a dual-energy X-ray absorptiometry (DXA scan).

Osteoporosis results in the increased risk of fracture. The majority of fractures are located in the lower extremities, with incidence up to 34% [45]. They have been found to occur while performing simple activities such as transfers, bed mobility, and self-care. The rotational movements that occur to the long bones of the legs during transfers or range of motion when completing self-care can result in torqueing of the bone, leading to fracture.

While dietary changes and the use of supplements can help slightly, the greatest impact on decreasing the severity of bone density, and in some circumstances improving bone density, is standing. Research exploring the benefits of standing has determined that the greatest benefit is in fact the improvement in bone density [46]. For this reason, standing will often occur in rehabilitation, with considerations for long-term use of a standing frame [47].

Neurogenic heterotopic ossification is another complication of spinal cord injury. It is characterized by the growth of new bone in the soft tissue surrounding a joint. This usually occurs in joints distal the spinal cord injury and is most commonly found in the hips and knees, though it has also been identified in elbows, hands, spine, ankles, and shoulders. The incidence ranges from 10 to 53% in persons with spinal cord injury [48]. It usually develops within the first 6 months post injury and can take 6–18 months to develop fully. The primary presentation is loss of range of motion, though pain can develop if the individual is sensate, spasticity can increase, and if the inflammation is intense enough, low-grade fevers can develop. It also often results in symptoms of autonomic dysreflexia. In worst cases, progression of the bone growth can become intertwined with neurovascular structures, impacting blood flow into an area.

Heterotopic ossification (HO) is an inflammatory process that occurs simultaneously to the increase in blood flow into the area around the joint. The area develops an increase in cellular and fibrous tissue growth, ultimately leading to the formation of osteoid material and the deposit of calcium. The cause is not entirely clear, but in some cases, there is found to be an increase in certain proteins. There is also a belief that damage to the sympathetic columns of the spinal cord can lead to the development of HO due to an imbalance in the autonomic nervous system. It is possible that trauma to the spinal cord near the sympathetic columns can lead to dysregulation here and dysautonomia. Another potential cause can be inflammation in the area due to pressure injury, thrombosis, or even excessive movement and tearing of tissue (Fig. 1.10).

The consequences of HO include loss of range of motion, pressure injury, and autonomic dysreflexia. Due to the growth of bone around the joint, flexibility is affected as ranging is interrupted by a bony block. It is important to note that loss of range is not due to a joint problem itself, but rather due to increased bone around the joint.

The loss of flexibility results in a shift in postural symmetry and increased pressure into weight-bearing surfaces. For individuals with HO, proper wheelchair seating and positioning become even more imperative. With loss of range of motion in the hip, the individual cannot sit upright to function. Forcing the person with heterotopic ossification to sit upright when they cannot results in a forceful movement of

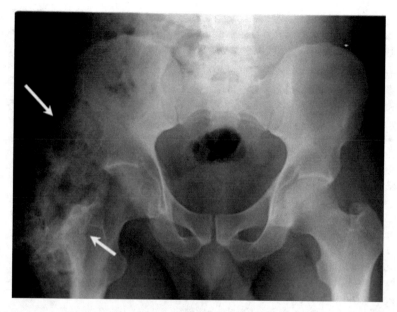

Fig. 1.10 X-ray of heterotopic ossification in the hip

the pelvis out of neutral, which leads to pressure and shear into all the weight-bearing tissues. It also leads to worsening overall alignment.

1.4.10   Cardiovascular Considerations

Cardiovascular disease (CVD) and stroke are higher among persons with SCI than those without SCI. Certain factors increase this risk, including decreased activity, irregularities in blood pressure, and chronic inflammation. Fluctuations between hypotension and hypertension from autonomic dysreflexia put added strain on the cardiovascular system, resulting in vascular injury and increasing the risks for CVD and stroke [49].

Deep vein thrombosis (DVT) and pulmonary embolism (PE) are complications associated with SCI. They're three times more likely to occur among persons with SCI as compared to the general population. Previous belief was that blood clots occur from pooling of blood in the lower extremities and the inability to use muscles in the legs to pump the fluid and blood back through the body. When blood pools, there is a greater risk for the development of a clot, resulting in a deep vein thrombosis or pulmonary embolism. Recent research indicates that paralysis and changes in neurologic function result in metabolic changes, which alter venous capacity and competence, increasing venous flow resistance.

The risk for development of DVT and thrombosis persists throughout the lifespan of the person with SCI due to these metabolic changes. Treatment of DVT and thrombosis has historically been using anticoagulants. But for this population, use of compression garments and pneumatic pumps in the legs and exercise are a better intervention to decrease risk of clot and thrombosis [50].

Resources
- Model System Knowledge Center
  msktc.org
- United Spinal Association
  unitedspinal.org
- Christopher and Dana Reeve Foundation
  christopherreeve.org
- National Pressure Injury Advisory Panel
  npiap.com
- CROWD: Center for Research on Women with Disabilities
  bcm.edu
- Office on Women's Health
  omenshealth.gov
- Primary Care and Spinal Cord Injury
  sci.washington.edu
- For Families Facing Spinal Cord Injuries
  FacingDisability.com
- American Academy of Physical Medicine and Rehabilitation

aapmr.org

References

1. White, N. H., & Black, N. H. (2017). *Spinal cord injury facts and figures at a glance. National Spinal Cord Injury Statistical Center, Facts and Figures at a Glance*. University of Alabama at Birmingham.
2. National Spinal Cord Injury Statistical Center (NSCIS) Facts and Figures at a Glance. (2016).
3. Witiw, C. D., & Fehlings, M. G. (2015). Acute spinal cord injury. *Journal of Spinal Disorders and Techniques, 28*(6), 202–210.
4. Wilson, J. R., Singh, A., Craven, C., Verrier, M. C., Drew, B., Ahn, H., Ford, M., & Fehlings, M. G. (2012). Early versus late surgery for traumatic spinal cord injury: The results of a prospective Canadian cohort study. *Spinal Cord, 50*(11), 840–843.
5. Sekhon, L. H., & Fehlings, M. G. (2001). Epidemiology, demographics, and pathophysiology of acute spinal cord injury. *Spine, 26*(24S), S2–S12.
6. NSCISC. (2011). *Annual report for the model spinal cord injury care systems*. N.S.C.I.S. Center.
7. Brienza, D., Krishnan, S., Karg, P., Sowa, G., & Allegretti, A. L. (2017). Predictors of pressure ulcer incidence following traumatic spinal cord injury: A secondary analysis of a prospective longitudinal study. *Spinal Cord, 56*(1), 28–34.
8. Bernhard, M., Gries, A., Kremer, P., & Böttiger, B. W. (2005). Spinal cord injury (SCI)—Prehospital management. *Resuscitation, 66*(2), 127–139.
9. Ahn, H., Singh, J., Nathens, A., MacDonald, R. D., Travers, A., Tallon, J., et al. (2011). Prehospital care management of a potential spinal cord injured patient: A systematic review of the literature and evidence-based guidelines. *Journal of Neurotrauma, 28*(8), 1341–1361.

10. Sheerin, F., & de Frein, R. (2007). The occipital and sacral pressures experienced by healthy volunteers under spinal immobilization: A trial of three surfaces. *Journal of Emergency Nursing, 33,* 447–450.

11. Kirshblum, S., & Eren, F. (2020). Anal reflex versus bulbocavernosus reflex in evaluation of patients with spinal cord injury. *Spinal Cord Series And Cases, 6*(1), 1–4.

12. Budisin, B., Bradbury, C. C., Sharma, B., Hitzig, S. L., Mikulis, D., Craven, C., et al. (2016). Traumatic brain injury in spinal cord injury: Frequency and risk factors. *Journal of Head Trauma Rehabilitation, 31*(4), E33–E42.

13. Wilson, J. R., Cadotte, D. W., & Fehlings, M. G. (2012). Clinical predictors of neurological outcome, functional status, and survival after traumatic spinal cord injury: A systematic review. *Journal of Neurosurgery: Spine, 17*(Suppl 1), 11–26.

14. Dvorak, M. F., Noonan, V. K., Fallah, N., Fisher, C. G., Finkelstein, J., Kwon, B. K., et al. (2015). The influence of time from injury to surgery on motor recovery and length of hospital stay in acute traumatic spinal cord injury: An observational Canadian cohort study. *Journal of Neurotrauma, 32*(9), 645–654.

15. Bellabarba, C., Fisher, C., Chapman, J. R., Dettori, J. R., & Norvell, D. C. (2010). Does early fracture fixation of thoracolumbar spine fractures decrease morbidity or mortality? *Spine, 35*(9S), S138–S145.

16. Berlly, M., & Shem, K. (2007). Respiratory management during the first five days after spinal cord injury. *Journal of Spinal Cord Medicine, 30*(4), 309–318.

17. Bono, C. M., & Heary, R. F. (2004). Gunshot wounds to the spine. *The Spine Journal, 4*(2), 230–240.

18. Garshick, E., Kelley, A., Cohen, S. A., Garrison, A., Tun, C. G., Gagnon, D., & Brown, R. (2005). A prospective assessment of mortality in chronic spinal cord injury. *Spinal Cord, 43*(7), 408–416.

19. Linn, W. S., Adkins, R. H., Gong, H., Jr., & Waters, R. L. (2000). Pulmonary function in chronic spinal cord injury: A cross-sectional survey of 222 southern California adult outpatients. *Archives of Physical Medicine and Rehabilitation, 81*(6), 757–763.

20. McKinley, W. O., Jackson, A. B., Cardenas, D. D., & Michael, J. (1999). Long-term medical complications after traumatic spinal cord injury: A regional model systems analysis. *Archives of Physical Medicine and Rehabilitation, 80*(11), 1402–1410.

21. Britton, D., Hoit, J. D., & Benditt, J. O. (2017, July). Dysarthria of spinal cord injury and its management. In *Seminars in speech and language* (Vol. 38, No. 03, pp. 161–172). Thieme Medical Publishers.

22. Edsberg, L. E., Black, J. M., Goldberg, M., McNichol, L., Moore, L., & Sieggreen, M. (2016). Revised national pressure ulcer advisory panel pressure injury staging system: Revised pressure injury staging system. *Journal of Wound, Ostomy, and Continence Nursing, 43*(6), 585–597.

23. Gefen, A., Brienza, D. M., Cuddigan, J., Haesler, E., & Kottner, J. (2022). Our contemporary understanding of the aetiology of pressure ulcers/pressure injuries. *International Wound Journal, 19*(3), 692–704.

24. McKinley, W. O., Gittler, M. S., Kirshblum, S. C., Stiens, S. A., & Groah, S. L. (2002). 2. Medical complications after spinal cord injury: Identification and management. *Archives of Physical Medicine and Rehabilitation, 83,* S58–S64, S90–S98.

25. Edsberg, L. E., Black, J. M., Goldberg, M., McNichol, L., Moore, L., & Sieggreen, M. (2016). Revised National Pressure Ulcer Advisory Panel pressure injury staging system: Revised pressure injury staging system. *Journal of Wound, Ostomy, and Continence Nursing, 43*(6), 585–597.

26. Richards, J. S., Waites, K., Chen, Y. Y., Kogos, S., & Schmitt, M. M. (2004). The epidemiology of secondary conditions following spinal cord injury. *Topics in Spinal Cord Injury Rehabilitation., 10*(1), 15–29.

27. Siddall, P. J., & Loeser, J. D. (2001). Pain following spinal cord injury. *Spinal Cord, 39*(2), 63–73.

28. Ehde, D. M., Jensen, M. P., Engel, J. M., Turner, J. A., Hoffman, A. J., & Cardenas, D. (2003). Chronic pain secondary to disability: A review. *Clinical Journal of Pain, 19*(3), 3–17.
29. Jensen, M. P., Hoffman, A. J., & Cardenas, D. D. (2005). Chronic pain in individuals with spinal cord injury: A survey and longitudinal study. *Spinal Cord, 43*(12), 704–712.
30. Cruz-Almeida, Y., Martinez-Arizala, A., & Widerström-Noga, E. (2005). Chronicity of pain associated with spinal cord injury: A longitudinal analysis. *Journal of Rehabilitation Research & Development, 42*(5), 585–594.
31. Littooij, E., Widdershoven, G. A., Stolwijk-Swüste, J. M., Doodeman, S., Leget, C. J., & Dekker, J. (2015). Global meaning in people with spinal cord injury: Content and changes. *The Journal of Spinal Cord Medicine., 39*(2), 197–205.
32. Paralyzed Veterans of America Consortium for Spinal Cord Medicine. (2005). Preservation of upper limb function following spinal cord injury: A clinical practice guideline for health-care professionals. *Journal of Spinal Cord Medicine, 28*(5), 434–470.
33. Sie, I. H., Waters, R. L., Adkins, R. H., & Gellman, H. (1992). Upper extremity pain in the postrehabilitation spinal cord injured patient. *Archives of Physical Medicine and Rehabilitation, 73*(1), 44–48.
34. Davies, A., Souza, L. H. D., & Frank, A. (2003). Changes in the quality of life in severely disabled people following provision of powered indoor/outdoor chairs. *Disability & Rehabilitation, 25*(6), 286–290.
35. Gorgey, A. S., Chiodo, A. E., Zemper, E. D., Hornyak, J. E., Rodriguez, G. M., & Gater, D. R. (2010). Relationship of spasticity to soft tissue body composition and the metabolic profile in persons with chronic motor complete spinal cord injury. *The Journal of Spinal Cord Medicine, 33*(1), 6–15.
36. Theriault, E. R., Huang, V., Whiteneck, G., Dijkers, M. P., & Harel, N. Y. (2018). Antispasmodic medications may be associated with reduced recovery during inpatient rehabilitation after traumatic spinal cord injury. *The Journal of Spinal Cord Medicine, 41*(1), 63–71.
37. Rabchevsky, A. G., & Kitzman, P. H. (2011). Latest approaches for the treatment of spasticity and autonomic dysreflexia in chronic spinal cord injury. *Neurotherapeutics, 8*(2), 274–282.
38. Ricciardi, R., Szabo, C. M., & Poullos, A. Y. (2007). Sexuality and spinal cord injury. *Nursing Clinics of North America, 42*(4), 675–684.
39. Brown, D. J., Hill, S. T., & Baker, H. W. (2006). Male fertility and sexual function after spinal cord injury. *Progress in Brain Research, 152*, 427–439.
40. Karlsson, A. K. (1999). Autonomic dysreflexia. *Spinal Cord, 37*(6), 383–391.
41. Munakata, M., Kameyama, J., Nunokawa, T., Ito, N., & Yoshinaga, K. (2001). Altered Mayer wave and baroreflex profiles in high spinal cord injury. *American Journal of Hypertension, 14*(2), 141–148.
42. Claydon, V. E., Steeves, J. D., & Krassioukov, A. (2006). Orthostatic hypotension following spinal cord injury: Understanding clinical pathophysiology. *Spinal Cord, 44*(6), 341–351.
43. Illman, A., Stiller, K., & Williams, M. (2000). The prevalence of orthostatic hypotension during physiotherapy treatment in patients with an acute spinal cord injury. *Spinal Cord, 38*(12), 741–747.
44. Middleton, J. W., Mann, L., & Leong, G. (2008). Management of spinal cord injury in general practice-part 1. *Australian Family Physician, 37*(4), 229.
45. Jiang, S. D., Dai, L. Y., & Jiang, L. S. (2006). Osteoporosis after spinal cord injury. *Osteoporosis International, 17*(2), 180–192.
46. Glickman, L. B., Geigle, P. R., & Paleg, G. S. (2010). A systematic review of supported standing programs. *Journal of Pediatric Rehabilitation Medicine, 3*(3), 197–213.
47. Dicianno, B. E., Morgan, A., Lieberman, J., & Rosen, L. (2013). RESNA position on the application of wheelchair standing devices: 2013 current state of the literature. Technical report, Rehabilitation Engineering and Assistive Technology.
48. Van Kuijk, A. A., Geurts, A. C. H., & Van Kuppevelt, H. J. M. (2002). Neurogenic heterotopic ossification in spinal cord injury. *Spinal Cord, 40*(7), 313–326.

49. Cragg, J. J., Noonan, V. K., Krassioukov, A., & Borisoff, J. (2013). Cardiovascular disease and spinal cord injury: Results from a national population health survey. *Neurology, 81*(8), 723–728.
50. Miranda, A. R., & Hassouna, H. I. (2000). Mechanisms of thrombosis in spinal cord injury. *Hematology/Oncology Clinics of North America, 14*(2), 401–416.

Chapter 2
Interventions

Rehabilitation of the person with spinal cord injury (SCI) is essential for improved function. Skilled intervention and the provision of custom complex rehabilitation technology allow for increased engagement and improved satisfaction with life.

2.1 Rehabilitation

Rehabilitation is a specialty that focuses on functional recovery. For persons with SCI, there exists a focused specialized service that provides even more attention to all aspects of SCI. The Spinal Cord Injury Model Systems (SCIMS) program began in 1970. SCIMS is sponsored by the National Institute on Disability, Independent Living, and Rehabilitation Research (NIDILRR) under the US Department of Health and Human Services (HHS).

SCIMS is a network of rehabilitation facilities that provides multidisciplinary care throughout the spectrum of injury. In order for these facilities to belong to SCIMS, they are required to provide care at all levels of intervention, from acute trauma to inpatient and outpatient rehabilitation, and include opportunities for vocational rehabilitation and lifetime follow-up. Each facility is required to keep data on the patients they serve; maintain this data with the National Spinal Cord Injury Database (NSCID), which was established in 1975; and engage in and disseminate research regarding the persons with SCI within their program [1].

Because of the SCIMS and subsequent NSCID, treatment of the person with SCI has evolved over time. Knowledge from research has identified effective assessment, intervention, and prevention. Due to the extensive experience in these facilities, it is highly recommended that the person with SCI undergoes rehabilitation there, if possible. While there are currently only 14 centers, there are other centers that provide exceptional intervention as well.

© The Author(s) 2022
J. Lieberman, *The Physical, Personal, and Social Impact of Spinal Cord Injury*,
SpringerBriefs in Public Health, https://doi.org/10.1007/978-3-031-18652-3_2

The rehabilitation team consists of the physiatrist, nursing care, neuropsychology, occupational therapy, physical therapy, social work, therapeutic recreation, speech and language pathology, and on occasion respiratory therapists.

- Physiatrist: This is the medical doctor specializing in rehabilitation. The physiatrist oversees the care of the person with SCI and is the leader of the medical team.
- Nurse: The nurse is an important part of the team to encourage not only carryover of daily activities to the unit but also education on bowel and bladder care.
- Neuropsychologist/psychologists: Provide counseling and educate on techniques to help with coping and adjustment after sustaining SCI.
- Occupational therapist (OT): Uses various techniques to improve and maintain performance of activities of daily living. This includes but is not limited to eating, dressing, bathing, home management, and transfers. The OT often works with the nurse on bowel and bladder management in the development of compensatory techniques when impaired hand function is present (with higher level SCI).
- Physical therapist (PT): Focuses on strength, range of motion, and endurance. During physical therapy, activities can also include tilt table use, transfers, mobility, and locomotion.
- Social worker (SW): Provides information and support to assist the transition out of the facility back home or to another residence, including skilled nursing facilities and sub-acute rehabilitation.
- Therapeutic recreation therapist: Uses certain activities to ease the return to everyday life, including outdoor excursions, socialization, etc.
- Speech therapist (ST): Can assist with problems of speech and swallowing, which can occur if there is limited diaphragm activity or if there is a history of intubation.
- Respiratory therapist: Can continue to be an active part of the team if the person with SCI is still on a ventilator.

The team works together when working with the person with SCI to develop a treatment plan. The treatment plan first identifies level of injury and completeness of injury, which is determined based upon the ASIA scale.

Spinal cord injuries are designated by complete or incomplete. A complete injury occurs when there is no movement or sensation below the level of injury. This is due to damage to the cord stopping the transfer of information between the brain and the body. An incomplete injury includes either sensory information or motor movement below the level of injury. This usually means that the damage has not interfered in transmission of all the information. The ASIA Impairment Scale (Fig. 2.1) was developed by the American Spinal Injury Association to clarify the extent of damage to the spinal cord. This is the predominant designation used in most hospitals and rehabilitation facilities. ASIA A is a complete injury, with complete loss of motor and sensation below the level of injury. ASIA B is an incomplete sensory injury, with complete loss of sensation below the level of injury but motor still present at some point below the level of injury. ASIA C is an incomplete motor injury. In this case there is still motor function below the level of injury, but more than half of the muscle groups below the level of injury are affected with no movement

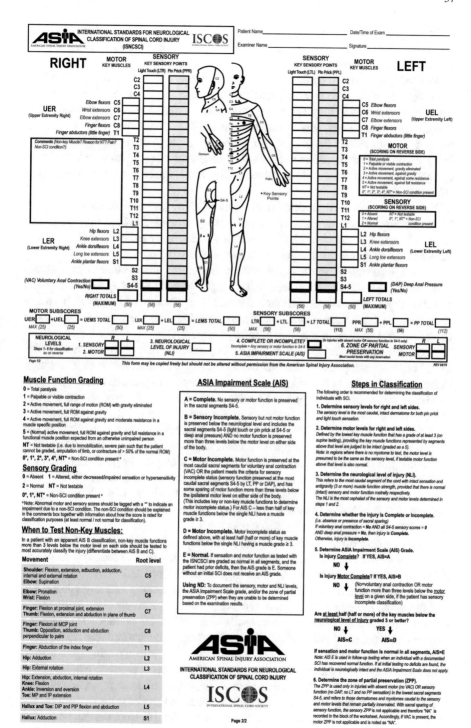

Fig. 2.1 ASIA scale, front and back

possible against gravity. ASIA D is similar to ASIA C, except here less than half the key muscle groups are affected against gravity. Finally, ASIA E is when motor and sensory function are normal.

Rehabilitation should occur the first day post injury [2]. During this stage, while the patient is still in the hospital, rehabilitation focuses on positioning to prevent contracture and pressure injury. During this time, the person with SCI is usually still experiencing acute secondary reactions from the SCI. Therapists will come to see the person with SCI at the bedside for treatment. If they are medically stable and there are no contraindications to do so, they might initiate activities such as sitting upright. However, this occurs more likely after transfer to inpatient acute rehabilitation.

Rate of recovery is dependent on the level of injury and completeness of injury. Motor incomplete has the greatest rate of recovery compared to motor complete and sensory incomplete injuries [3]. Rates of motor and sensory recovery are believed to decrease within 6 months to a year after initial injury [4].

Once transferred to acute rehabilitation, the entire team becomes part of the treatment plan with the person with SCI. The person with SCI is evaluated by each member of the team to determine their functional capabilities and to develop a treatment plan. Each treatment plan is specific to the individual. There are however some considerations specific to the level of injury (Table 2.1).

With this in mind, each service begins to generate goals with the person with SCI. The team and person with SCI must work closely together when generating these goals for them to be achievable. Patients are able to achieve meaningful performance when they feel supported by the team of healthcare professionals. They are also better able to fight to achieve success with their goals if they are matched with the professionals [5]. This reinforces the need for the team to work with the person with SCI. When not supported, there is greater likelihood the person with SCI will fight back against the team and either not engage or perform their own activities. Goals are designed to be achievable and can be modified as there is progression or regression during the rehabilitation stay. Goals are not only for the person with SCI to achieve, but goals also consist of the person with SCI being able to direct others to assist them with their care.

Rehabilitation often focuses on compensation and compensatory techniques. This is due to the expectation that there will not be full motor and sensory recovery. Skills addressed during therapy are learning new techniques to dress, transfer, bathe, prepare food, move around in bed, and manage a wheelchair and any other goals specific to the individual. This occurs by breaking down activities into manageable tasks for the patient to achieve success within their level of function. Learning requires repetition and practice to be able to problem solve performance in all environments. Repetition has been found to result in motor recovery, which can lead to improved recovery of function for the person with SCI. This is due to what is called activity-dependent plasticity. Activity-based therapy consists of repetition of task, which in turn can retrain the nervous system to recover motor tasks [6]. This is the concept behind locomotion training with external skeletal devices but can be carried over to therapy-focused activities of daily living.

Table 2.1 Level of injury functional status, goals, and equipment needs

Level of injury/expected motor control	Functional capabilities	Goals	Equipment needs
C2–C3: Limited head and neck movement	Breathing: Depends on a ventilator Communication: Can be limited or impossible Self-care: dependent Transfers: dependent	Wheelchair mobility: Independent with power wheelchair Independent pressure relief in power wheelchair Independent communication Independent control of environmental technology including, but not limited to, TV, doors, lights, appliances	Suction machine Ventilator with backup battery and generator in the event of power loss Possible phrenic pacemaker Speech generating device if communication is impaired Sip and puff attendant call switch Mouth stick to access various technology, including tablets and smart phone Eye gaze for computer access If speech is normal, voice-activated computer access and environmental control Environment control: smart hubs, switches, and infrared, Bluetooth and cloud-based technology Power wheelchair with power seat functions and supportive and pressure relieving seating system Mechanical transfer system (Hoyer): floor or ceiling based
C4: Shoulder shrug	Breathing: may initially need a ventilator Communication: normal Self-care: full assistance Transfers: dependent	Wheelchair mobility: independent with power wheelchair Independent pressure relief in power wheelchair Independent communication Independent control of environmental technology including, but not limited to, TV, doors, lights, appliances	Cough assist Environment control: smart hubs, switches, and infrared, Bluetooth and cloud-based technology Power wheelchair with power seat functions and supportive and pressure relieving seating system Mechanical transfer system (Hoyer): floor or ceiling based

(continued)

Table 2.1 (continued)

Level of injury/ expected motor control	Functional capabilities	Goals	Equipment needs
C5: Elbow flexion, forearm supination	Breathing: may initially need cough assist for management of secretions Self-care: some assistance Transfers: minimal to maximal assistance	Wheelchair mobility: independent with power wheelchair Some potential for independent mobility with manual wheelchair with projection rims Independent pressure relief in power wheelchair Independent control of environmental technology including, but not limited to, TV, doors, lights, appliances Self-care: eating and some grooming: independent with set-up with adaptive device Dressing: upper body can be independent after set-up Bathing: can perform some independently with devices and after set-up Bowel and bladder: Dependent: Pressure relief: independent with power seating; may be partially independent with forward and sideways lean	Power wheelchair with power seat functions and supportive and pressure relieving seating system Manual wheelchair with handrim projections Environment control: smart hubs, switches, and infrared, Bluetooth and cloud-based technology Hand and wrist cuff to hold utensils, grooming tools (toothbrush, razor, makeup brush, etc.), and sponge for bathing Cup with handle, long flexible straw Bladder: Can be independent with electric leg bag opener Assistance with sliding board transfers Driving evaluation for hand controls

C6: Forearm supination and pronation, wrist extension	Self-care: initially assisted Transfers: initially dependent Mobility: initially dependent Bowel and bladder: initially dependent	Self-care: independent after set-up with adaptive devices, except assistance for lower body dressing and bathing. Bowel and bladder: independence with devices is possible Transfers: independent Mobility: independent with power wheelchair; potential for independence with manual wheelchair with projection rims Pressure relief: independent with power seating; may be partially independent with forward and sideways lean forward and sideways lean	Power wheelchair with power seat functions and supportive and pressure relieving seating system Manual wheelchair with handrim projections Environment control: smart hubs, switches, and infrared, Bluetooth and cloud-based technology Hand and wrist cuff to hold utensils, grooming tools (toothbrush, razor, makeup brush, etc.), and sponge for bathing Cup with handle, long flexible straw Bladder: Can be independent with electric leg bag opener Assistance with sliding board transfers Driving evaluation for hand controls
C7: ability to extend elbow	Self-care: initially assisted Transfers: initially assisted Mobility: initially assisted Bowel and bladder: initially assisted	Self-care: fully independent except may still need assistance for lower body dressing Bowel and bladder: independent with devices Transfers: independent Mobility: independent with manual wheelchair Pressure relief: independent with forward and sideways lean	Padded transfer tub bench Padded commode for independent access during bowel and bladder Ultralight manual wheelchair with supportive and pressure relieving seating system Devices for self-care: reacher, long handled dressing stick, long handled sponge for bathing, zipper pull, long shoehorn Bowel and bladder: leg spreader, suppository inserter, adaptive mirror Driving evaluation for hand controls

(continued)

Table 2.1 (continued)

Level of injury/ expected motor control	Functional capabilities	Goals	Equipment needs
C8–T1: hand and finger movement	Self-care: initially assisted Transfers: initially assisted Mobility: initially assisted Bowel and bladder: initially assisted	Self-care: fully independent. Might still need adaptive devices Bowel and bladder: independent with devices Transfers: independent Mobility: independent with manual wheelchair Pressure relief: independent with forward and sideways lean	Padded transfer tub bench Padded commode for independent access during bowel and bladder Ultralight manual wheelchair with supportive and pressure relieving seating system Driving evaluation for hand controls
T2–L1: Trunk control due to increased innervation of chest and abdominal muscles	Self-care: initially assisted Transfers: initially assisted Mobility: initially assisted	Full independence with self-care Bowel and bladder: independent Full independence with transfers Full independence with propulsion Pressure relief: independent with forward and sideways lean	Padded transfer tub bench Padded commode for independent access during bowel and bladder Ultralight manual wheelchair with supportive and pressure relieving seating system Driving evaluation for hand controls
L2–S1: Movement of hips, knees and ankles	Independent self-care Independent transfers Independent with propulsion Possibility for independent walking	Full independence with all self-care and mobility Bowel and bladder: independent Full independence with transfers Full independence with propulsion Pressure relief: independent with forward and sideways lean	Ultralight manual wheelchair with supportive and pressure relieving seating system Leg braces from hip to foot with walker of crutches

When creating a treatment plan with goals, it is important that the activities are challenging but doable. One way to approach treatment planning is creating a flow state. Flow explores the idea of intrinsic motivation. The idea behind being in a flow state is to engage in activities that are just challenging enough and manageable to sustain focus. When the activity is too challenging, anxiety creeps in, and the person loses focus or a desire to engage. When the activity is not challenging enough, the person becomes bored and loses focus or a desire to engage [7].

While the treatment provided varies from person to person, there are certain consistencies among interventions for persons with SCI. The largest focus is found to be on performance of activities of daily living (ADL) and on range of motion and strengthening. For persons with tetraplegia, a focus is on strengthening the tenodesis for function [8]. Because tenodesis is essential for task performance, there should be attention paid to promoting it. This can be done through orthotics and straps.

The OT and PT will also address access in the home and community, including accessing rooms of the home, as well as entering and exiting the home and building. Education on adaptations and rights under the Americans with Disabilities Act should occur. Depending on the level of injury, recommendations for assistive technology occur based upon assessment of need. This can include home access and computer access. If the person with SCI has tenodesis, splinting can occur to promote this prehension pattern. The OT and PT are also the primary members of the team when assessing for wheelchair use, both manual and powered mobility.

Length of stay in the hospital and in acute rehabilitation has changed since 1970, when statistics were initially gathered. Hospital stay has declined from 24 to 11 days, and acute rehabilitation has declined from 98 to 31 days [9]. Persons with paraplegia are hospitalized on average for less time than persons with tetraplegia. Due to shortened length of stay, after acute rehabilitation the person with SCI is often discharged to sub-acute rehabilitation (SAR) for continued intervention.

After acute rehabilitation, there are two possible options for discharge: home to the community to participate in outpatient rehabilitation or to a SAR facility. Persons with SCI who participate in acute rehabilitation are more likely to return home to the community and then those who do not participate in acute rehabilitation [10]. In addition to lack of participation in acute rehabilitation after SCI, another factor that impacts discharge to home is access. Environmental factors, including steps and doorway widths that do not allow for wheelchair use, can result in discharge to SAR. While participating in therapy in SAR, the person with SCI can be awaiting modifications to their existing home or a wheelchair-accessible apartment. Length of stay can be dependent on these factors. The person with SCI participates in daily therapies, but for a lesser amount of time than while they were participating in acute rehabilitation.

On some occasions, after the person with SCI is discharged home, they will receive home therapies while they prepare for outpatient therapy. Circumstances can be that the person is not stable enough to travel into the community to participate in therapies yet that they are awaiting insurance authorization to participate in outpatient therapies or that there is a waiting list for outpatient therapy services.

Outpatient therapy involves traveling to a clinic in the community. The amount of therapy can vary, with some persons with SCI participating in outpatient services up to 18 months. Participation is often dependent on reimbursement by insurance for the services providing care, including OT and PT. Due to the specific needs of the person with SCI, there should be an attempt made to participate in therapy that is designed for treatment to the person with SCI. The needs for intervention are more extensive than the person with an alternative disability, and as such the person with SCI should engage in therapies with clinicians who are experienced with working the SCI population.

2.2   Wheelchairs and Complex Rehab Technology

Wheelchair use is a significant component for participation in daily activities and in life for the person with SCI. Therefore, it is imperative that the wheelchair is properly fitted to the user. A poorly fit wheelchair can result in pain, deformity, and pressure injury. A properly designed wheelchair will promote function, encourage postural alignment towards neutral, provide proper pressure distribution, and limit complaints of pain. For this reason, it is essential the person with SCI is evaluated by a team that specializes in wheelchair seating, positioning, and mobility. Most rehabilitation facilities have a wheelchair clinic where this assessment can occur. To find a wheelchair clinic near you, you can contact local facilities or local spinal cord support groups.

There are several members of the team involved in the assessment: the person with SCI, their caretakers, the medical team (therapist and physician), the rehabilitation technology supplier, and the insurance plan. Here we will explore the stages of wheelchair assessment, acquisition, and use.

2.2.1   The Assessment Process

There are several components to a proper assessment. A thorough history taking is important in order to understand the individual's medical, personal, and environmental needs. This includes a review of the medical chart and an interview with the person with SCI and their caretakers.

2.2.1.1   The Physical Assessment

The assessment can occur at various times: while still in acute rehabilitation, upon discharge, or many years down the road when acquiring a new wheelchair. The needs at these different stages can change as well. Newly injured individuals usually have less skills than those many years post injury. For this reason, it is important to match the technology to the user to ensure success. This requires a thorough understanding of their physical and emotional needs. We will discuss the subjective experience of wheelchair use in Chap. 3. But it is important to understand as the physical evaluation begins that a variety of emotions can come out during this assessment process. Individuals who have sustained SCI are often focused on the goal of walking [11], so they may not be full participants in the evaluation process. Furthermore, they may desire a device that feels less "disabling" and focus on something that may not clinically be the best long-term solution [12].

There are several stages to the assessment of wheelchair need. The assessment begins with understanding how the person with SCI sits. There are three types of seated postures to consider when determining the amount of support necessary to provide the person with SCI when seated in the wheelchair (Table 2.2).

The physical assessment consists of both a seated and supine assessment. The person is first assessed supine. This allows for true postural assessment with the removal of gravity. The patient lies down on a mat. Postural alignment and range of motion are assessed to determine flexibility of the asymmetry and joint mobility. The pelvic position is assessed, looking for any asymmetries including obliquity (designated by the lower side), rotation, and tilt. The spinal position is also assessed, looking for scoliosis (lateral trunk flexion), a flat lumbar space, or a kyphosis ("rounded back").

After assessing spinal position, lower extremity range of motion is examined, looking for flexibility of the hip and knee toward neutral. Because the muscles that perform these movements cross joints, their flexibility needs to be explored as pull can alter the position of the pelvis. For example, the muscles behind the upper leg (the hamstrings) are secured to the bones below the knee and above the hip (the pelvis). Flexion or extension at one joint impacts flexion or extension at the other joint. If hamstrings are tight, extending the knee beyond its allowable range will extend the hip and pull on the pelvis, moving it out of neutral.

HO in the hips can limit flexion or extension due to the buildup of bone on either side of the joint. It most commonly results in extensions. With HO there is a higher risk for pressure injury from shearing as the body repositions itself. This risk is located at the bony prominence along the seated surface and the plantar aspect of the feet from force into footplates. HO in the knees can impact foot support if the limitations are in flexion or extension. On some occasions HO can interfere so much in the seated posture and in skin health that patients will be referred to orthopedics for surgical evaluation.

After the supine assessment occurs, a seated assessment occurs, looking at the same pelvic and spinal postures examined while supine. Measurements are taken while seated with as much elongation as possible to ensure proper fit. One of the

Table 2.2 Seated postures

Hands free	Able can sit unsupported up against gravity
Hands dependent	Rely on at least one hand to maintain upright
Prop sitter	Require extensive support to remain upright against gravity

goals of proper sitting is equal pressure distribution. Understanding how much force is needed to support posture and move asymmetry toward mid-line is important and can only be determined by doing the hands-on assessment.

The assessment also examines skin integrity and the presence of pressure injuries or scar from the initial trauma, sensation, continence, alignment, and balance. Pain is an important part of the assessment, identifying if the cause is neuropathic or musculoskeletal. Back pain is often located in the lumbar spine and can often be relieved with 10 degrees of extension and lumbar support. Upper trapezium and levator scapulae pain is common because of scapular protraction and elevation, which are associated with a thoracic kyphosis. Upper extremity pain is often postural due to poor alignment. Kyphosis results in a collapsed posture, with scapular protraction and elevation. This causes impingement into the front of the shoulder. This can be addressed by altering the center of gravity of the wheelchair, affecting rear wheel placement, and creating dump (when the front of the wheelchair seat is higher than the rear). The goal is for the middle finger to be in close proximity to the hub of the rear wheel. This allows for more fluid strides with less frequency of repetition [13].

Other considerations are as follows:

Range of motion and strength: This will determine ability to self-propel.
Diagnoses: Are there additional diagnoses to take into consideration. This can include cardiac and respiratory disease, which can affect endurance and the ability to propel, and arthritis, which can lead to greater risk of pain and injury.
Postural stability and balance: This can narrow down frame setup or the need for power over manual wheelchair.
Age: This can narrow down manual versus powered mobility.

Considerations for paraplegia are a manual wheelchair unless there is presence of upper limb dysfunction, severe postural deformity, pressure ulcer, or cardiac and respiratory issues. Pain, pressure injury, and deformity are the main symptoms that limit the recommendation of a manual wheelchair for full-time propulsion.

Considerations for tetraplegia are a power wheelchair unless there is functional hand use or issues of access. The lower the level of injury, the greater the option for use of a manual wheelchair with this population.

2.2.1.2   The Social and Environmental Assessment

While the physical assessment gives the bulk of the data in equipment selection, there are several other very important areas to explore with the person with SCI. The home environment is important to assess. Considerations are entryway steps and hallway and doorway widths. It is not always possible to match the technology to the environment, but it must be considered. For example, a power wheelchair cannot easily be carried up steps since they can weigh up to 400 pounds. Likewise, the overall width of the equipment cannot always be modified. Manual wheelchair overall base widths are the measurement of the desired width match to the person's hip width and the wheels, while power wheelchairs have a fixed overall base width. Certain locations are harder to access than others, including bathrooms. In urban areas bathroom doorway widths average 21″. Doorway measurements and floor-plans are often part of the home assessment provided while on the acute rehabilitation unit, as well as when pursuing new equipment down the road.

Another consideration is work, school, or leisure activities. Not only are overall dimensions important in all environments, but here environmental access is examined. For example, what form of transportation is being used to access the community and work settings (i.e., car, bus, train, subway). This can impact the overall design of the equipment selected.

Roles and responsibilities are also important to explore. The parent with SCI may have to carry their child during propulsion. The student with SCI may have to carry books and supplies. How these different needs are going to be met can impact equipment design.

2.2.2 Considerations for Wheelchair Design: Manual Wheelchair

Manual wheelchairs can come in two designs: rigid and folding. Rigid frame wheelchairs (Fig. 2.2) often allow for more efficient propulsion due to fewer moving parts and lighter weight, but they don't disassemble as easily as folding frame wheelchairs (Fig. 2.3). These disassemble by folding down the seat back and taking off the wheels to create a smaller package. Folding frame wheelchairs (Fig 2.3) are easier to transport but can be heavier, and, because they shift a little more, they are not as efficient.

Some persons with SCI may not be ready for sitting in a rigid or folding frame wheelchair and lack the ability to control a power wheelchair. Another possibility is they require positional change but reside in an inaccessible environment with steps. Under these circumstances they may be provided with a manual reclining wheelchair or manual tilt in space wheelchair. In a manual reclining wheelchair, the back folds down and can be raised back up. This is good for management of orthostasis but results in shear along the seated surface and is not a good long-term option. The other option, the manual tilt in space wheelchair (Fig. 2.4}, results in tipping the entire seat backward. This can also be used to manage orthostasis but results in less shear along the seated surface.

The weight of the wheelchair is an important consideration. Various materials are used now in fabrication, including aluminum, titanium, and carbon fiber. Aluminum is the most commonly used material. The lighter-weight materials are often not reimbursed by insurance. Medicare classifies wheelchairs by their weight (Table 2.3).

Persons with SCI below C6 are appropriate for a K0005 manual wheelchair. There are however some occasions where persons with C6 are appropriate for management of a K0005 manual wheelchair. This should be based upon assessment and trial. The lighter-weight wheelchair results in the need for less force during

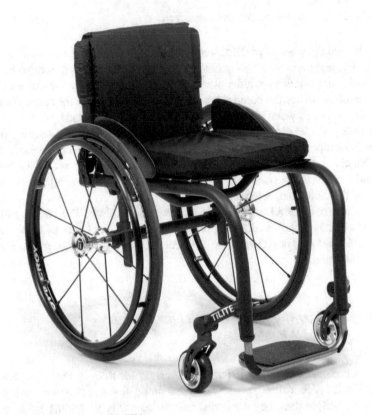

Fig. 2.2 Rigid frame wheelchair; TiLite

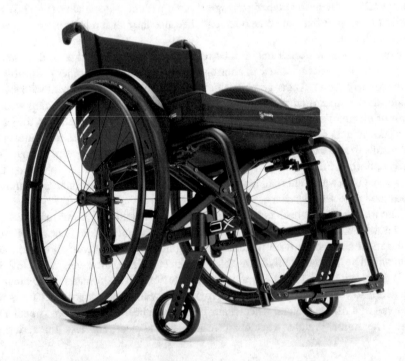

Fig. 2.3 Folding frame wheelchair; KiMobility

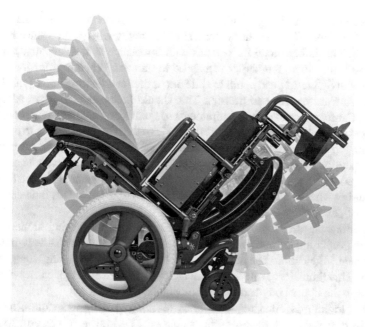

Fig. 2.4 Manual tilt in space wheelchair; KiMobility

Table 2.3 Medicare manual wheelchair codes

K0001	Standard manual wheelchair; weighs 35 pounds or more
K0002	Standard manual wheelchair with a height (17″ to 18″)
K0003	Lightweight wheelchair
K0004	High strength lightweight wheelchair; weighs 30–35 pounds
K0005	Ultra-lightweight wheelchair; weighs under 30 pounds

propulsion due to decreased roll resistance. The heavier the base is, the greater the resistance is, and the harder it is to push. Therefore, it is important that persons with SCI use as lightweight a wheelchair as possible. In addition, persons with SCI require greater adjustability in their wheel placement and seat and back angles due to multiple factors, including imbalance, tone, range of motion, and strength. There is a lot of research supporting the idea that wheel location and access are imperative for prevention of upper limb dysfunction [13]. For example, the rear wheel should be as far forward as possible without impacting stability. Wheel access requires that when the user places their hand on the top of the wheel, the angle between the upper arm and forearm is between 100 and 120 degrees.

There are several additional considerations for fit. Width is important. If the wheelchair is too narrow, it will create increased pressure into the hips and can result in impairment in skin integrity. If the seat is too wide, the wheels are farther away, and greater strain is placed on the upper extremities during propulsion. Seat slope is another consideration. This is the difference between the front and rear heights in relation to the ground. The greater the difference between the two, the greater the slope. Slope can allow for a shift in gravity when seated since it creates static tilt. This is beneficial for persons with imbalance and asymmetry. However, the greater the slope, the harder it may be to transfer. When transferring out, the person with SCI must push uphill to slide out of the seat, fighting gravity, as they try to move toward the edge to transfer. This should be considered when addressing design. Camber is one of the requirements to qualify for a K0005 under Medicare and most other insurances. Camber is the angle of the wheel in relation to the frame, with the top being closer and the base being wider. Camber can create increased frame stability. The greater the camber, the wider the base width, which needs to be considered for access. Significant increases in camber are generally added to frames used during wheelchair sports since this creates a stable base. This includes tennis, basketball, and rugby.

Providing an ultra-lightweight wheelchair with proper seating alone will not result in proper upper limb function. Propulsion technique is also a very important component. Education on propulsion techniques includes using long smooth strokes. This limits force into the wheel and repetition. Repetition causes increased strain into the upper body and increased complaints of pain.

Skills training is often required when teaching specific techniques, including maneuvering various surfaces, curbs, stairs, etc., as well as to perform wheelies. Many spinal cord rehabilitation programs have a wheelchair skills class. Initial skills training consists of moving forward, backward, and side to side. From there, more advanced skills are taught, including managing curbs, wheelies, and stairs.

2.2.2.1   Manual Wheelchair Components

The wheelchair consists of several accessory components. While they all are important, there are certain accessory components that require greater consideration when working with the person with SCI:

Tires: the most common type is pneumatic, which is air filled. These can come in different designs, including standard pneumatic tires and high-pressure tires, which resemble bicycle tires. These are lighter in weight and provide greater shock absorption. These can puncture and require maintenance. The better they are maintained, the less likely they will puncture. The alternative designs that do not puncture are solid tires and pneumatic tires with foam-filled inserts. These are both heavier than pneumatic tires. Solid tires are the least costly, but the most uncomfortable since they provide absolutely no suspension. Suspension is an important consideration for persons with spasticity and pain. The firmer the ride, the greater the complaints of pain and the increased trigger of spasticity, which impacts alignment and wheel access.

Wheels: Wheels can come with plastic spokes, metal spokes, or composite spokes. The spokes are what connect the tire to the wheel hub and secure the wheel to the wheelchair. Plastic spokes, also known as mag tires, are the easiest to maintain.

They are however quite a bit heavier. Metal spokes are lighter, but require some maintenance, with the spokes loosening or snapping over time. Composite spokes have greater suspension and are more durable. They are much harder to damage. They are however quite costly and are not always reimbursed by insurance.

Casters: Casters are the smaller wheels in the front of the wheelchair frame. They can be of various sizes in height and width. The larger the wheels are in height and the wider they are, the greater obstacles they can travel over. The smaller they are, the easier to propel since there is less rolling resistance due to a smaller base size.

Push rims: Push rims can be aluminum or covered in a material that creates friction for greater push for those with impaired hand function. They can also have protrusions to push off of for those with greater impairment in prehension. Some rims are oblong to create a more ergonomic position for the wrist and hand when grasping the wheel and propelling. These are ideal for persons with hand and wrist pain.

Armrests: Armrests are a very important part of the wheelchair in the role they play with transfers, weight shift, and function. They can be easily swung aside, as in tubular armrests, or flipped back, adjustable in height, or shorter and longer, as in desk or full-length style. Having knowledge as to how the person with SCI will complete these functions in the wheelchair is important when deciding which armrest will be best.

Footrests: Rigid frame wheelchairs have either a platform, rigid or flip back, or plates that can flip out to the side. The consideration is how the person with SCI transfers. Flip back options are pursued if the transfers require both feet be on the floor or if the person with SCI is using leg braces. These are heavier and can loosen over time, but they can allow for safer squat pivot transfers rather than standing on the platform. Folding frame wheelchairs have footrests that swing out to the side or under the seat.

Wheel locks: Wheel locks secure the wheelchair when not propelling. There are ones located on the side of the frame in front of the wheels that either push forward or pull back to lock. There is also an option that is located under the seat, so the wheel locks are not in the way during propulsion.

2.2.3 Considerations for Wheelchair Design: Power Wheelchair

A power wheelchair is recommended for persons with SCI who are either unable to self-propel, who have developed strain in their upper body that impacts function (including transfers and mobility), or who have developed significant impairment in skin integrity with pressure injuries and are unable to shift their own weight.

Power wheelchairs have three primary classifications for base design: front (Fig. 2.5), mid- (Fig. 2.6), and rear wheel drive (Fig. 2.7). This determines where the larger wheel is located. The decision for the selection of the drive configuration is based upon the environments the wheelchair will be used in. Front wheel drive chairs have the larger wheel in the front of the base, ahead of the user's center of gravity. They are able to climb over thresholds and uneven terrain better and have a very tight turning radius. Mid-wheel drive chairs have the larger wheel directly underneath the user's center of gravity. This results in the smallest turning radius. However, the casters are more likely to get caught in holes and divots. As a result, this base is better for use indoors. And finally, rear wheel drive wheelchairs have the rear wheel behind the user with a larger center of gravity. This results in a larger turning radius but greater stability. They can also be tipped back when traveling over a larger threshold or step.

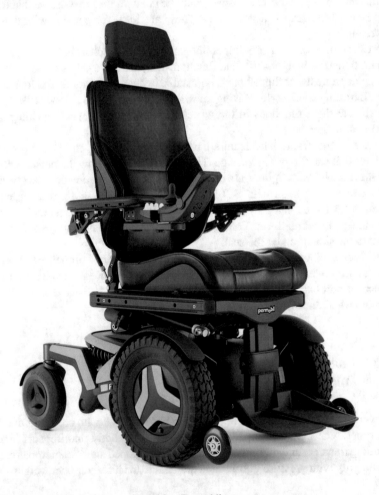

Fig. 2.5 Power wheelchair, front wheel drive; Permobil

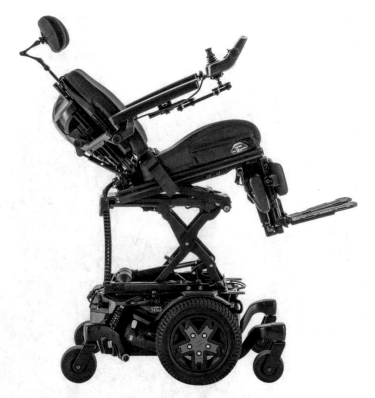

Fig. 2.6 Power wheelchair, mid-wheel drive; Quantum Rehab

2.2.3.1   Power Assist Wheelchairs

Power assist wheelchairs (PAW) are manual wheelchairs with a motor that supplements push. The motor can be attached to the camber bar or axle plate or located in the rear wheels. The models that attach to the camber or axle plate are easily removed, allowing for use of the wheelchair without or with power without adding weight to the frame. This allows for an easier transition from manual to power (Figs. 2.8 and 2.9). Those motors located in the rear wheel are either controlled via pushing on the rim or through a joystick attached to the armrest. These are harder to disassemble as there is always a component to the product secured to the frame. As such, when propelling without power, there is still added weight.

PAW provide two possibilities. They provide for an option to have both power and manual operation, allowing for manual propulsion and then adding on the power component when either going a long distance or when fatigued and needing additional assistance. They also allow for the use of a motorized device for persons with steps to enter their residence. Motorized wheelchair can weigh up to 400 pounds. For persons with steps to enter their residence, this is not a realistic option for access. PAW allow for a motorized option that can more easily be transported up stairs. However, because the base is a manual wheelchair, this is not as durable

Fig. 2.7 Power
wheelchair, rear wheel
drive; Invacare

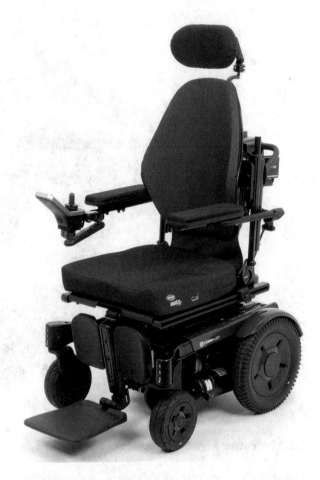

Fig. 2.8 Power assist
wheelchair on chair,
SmartDrive; Permobil

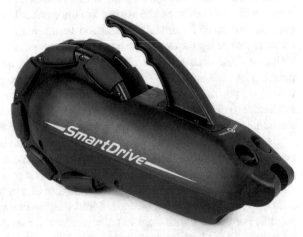

Fig. 2.7 Power wheelchair, rear wheel drive; Invacare

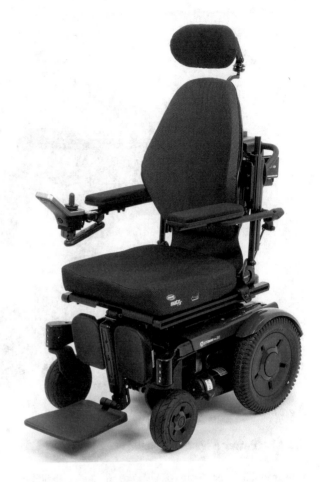

Fig. 2.8 Power assist wheelchair on chair, SmartDrive; Permobil

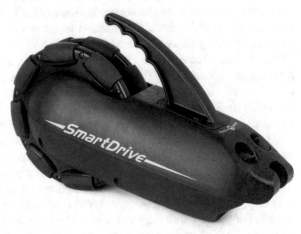

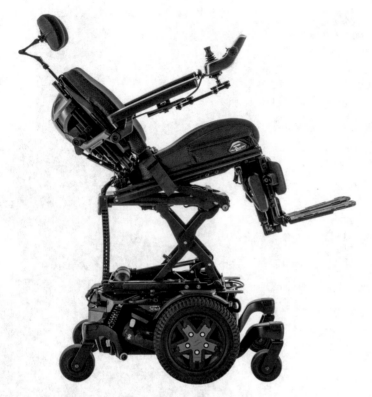

Fig. 2.6 Power wheelchair, mid-wheel drive; Quantum Rehab

2.2.3.1 Power Assist Wheelchairs

Power assist wheelchairs (PAW) are manual wheelchairs with a motor that supplements push. The motor can be attached to the camber bar or axle plate or located in the rear wheels. The models that attach to the camber or axle plate are easily removed, allowing for use of the wheelchair without or with power without adding weight to the frame. This allows for an easier transition from manual to power (Figs. 2.8 and 2.9). Those motors located in the rear wheel are either controlled via pushing on the rim or through a joystick attached to the armrest. These are harder to disassemble as there is always a component to the product secured to the frame. As such, when propelling without power, there is still added weight.

PAW provide two possibilities. They provide for an option to have both power and manual operation, allowing for manual propulsion and then adding on the power component when either going a long distance or when fatigued and needing additional assistance. They also allow for the use of a motorized device for persons with steps to enter their residence. Motorized wheelchair can weigh up to 400 pounds. For persons with steps to enter their residence, this is not a realistic option for access. PAW allow for a motorized option that can more easily be transported up stairs. However, because the base is a manual wheelchair, this is not as durable

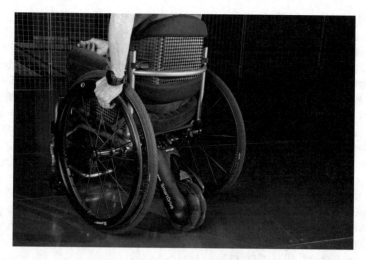

Fig. 2.9 Power assist wheelchair off chair, SmartDrive; Permobil

outdoors when used with the motor. Considerations are for terrain and the effect of power over time on the frame and casters.

Another consideration is insurance reimbursement. Medicare will only cover PAW if the beneficiary requires powered mobility full time in the home for performance of mobility-related activities of daily living and they have been utilizing a manual wheelchair for 1 year prior to consideration of PAW.

2.2.3.2   Power Seat Functions

Power wheelchairs allow for the addition of power seat functions. There are several different options that exist. For persons with higher-level injuries or persons with pressure injuries and orthostatic hypotension, power seat functions are essential.

Power tilt: Tilt is when the seat and back move together, allowing the seat to go all the way back and come back upright. There is decreased risk of shear when changing one's position. Tilting backward more than 25 degrees can allow for some reduction in pressure along the seated surface.

Power recline: Recline is when just the back moves in relation to the seat. Recline can be beneficial for persons with limitations in hip range of motion due to heterotopic ossification, since it allows for an open seat to back angle to accommodate to hip range of motion through recline while also allowing for the back to come up for completion of functional activities at a tabletop. Recline also allows for opening the back during catheterization and bowel and bladder management for greater access. However, lowering and raising the back alone can result in shear along the back and seated surface, which is detrimental for persons with pressure injuries or those at high risk for pressure injuries.

Power tilt and power recline: Research indicates that the greatest reductions in pressure are seen when tilt and recline are used together, either at tilt of 35° with recline 100° or tilt of 15–25° with recline of 120° [14]. For persons with SCI, the combination of power tilt and recline is usually recommended given the multiple secondary complications associated with SCI Figs. 2.10.

Power elevating legrests: Allow for a change on knee and foot angle in relation to the seat. This allows for flexion and extension at the knee. Some legrests can articulate during movement, which allows for lengthening at the knee and decreases the impact on the hip. These are better able to support spasticity in the lower extremities, allowing for dynamic positional change as spasm is triggered. They are also best able to manage edema, when used with tilt and recline, due to the ability to raise the foot 30 cm above the heart. There are two options for foot support: a platform or separate footrests. Both can elevate fully, with the separate footrests having the option to move independently. The platform is the most frequently selected option as it allows for feet to be tucked back farther and results in a smaller overall turning radius.

Seat elevation: The seat elevator raises and lowers the seat height while the user is seated. Seat elevation can benefit reach, facilitate transfers, enhance orientation, and promote social engagement. Research has shown that wheelchair users perform more overhead activities than those who do not use wheelchairs. Research also shows that there is a strong correlation with overhead reach and shoulder pain [15, 16]. The use of a power elevating seat can limit overhead activities and in turn limit upper body strain. Persons with SCI can only enter and exit their wheelchair by transferring. Some research indicates that transfers can occur up to 20 times a day. The force applied into the shoulder when pushing down during transfers is extremely high and places the individual at higher rates of shoulder problems [17]. Raising the overall height decreases the forces into the shoulder when transferring and in turn can decrease upper limb dysfunction and pain. Power seat elevation however is not reimbursed by most insurance plans, including Medicare, as it is considered a non-covered item. However, most manufacturers offer grants to cover the cost. Application for the grant requires a letter of need written by the person with SCI (Fig. 2.11).

Power standing: A power standing device is a power wheelchair with the capability of bringing the user up to a standing position. There are two types of standing possible with a power standing wheelchair: sit to stand or tilt table. These position the user in different postures as they come up to stand. This can be beneficial in decreasing the incidence of orthostatic hypotension. Power standing devices can be used to improve range of motion and decrease the risk of contracture through movement, promote bone health through weight bearing, reduce spasticity through weight bearing, improve bowel and bladder function through postural positioning, promote vital organ capacity through postural positioning, improve circulation through postural positioning, decrease the incidence of pressure injury through offloading, promote function, and improve quality of life and perception of self. Like the power seat elevator, this is often not covered by most insurances, including Medicare (Fig. 2.12).

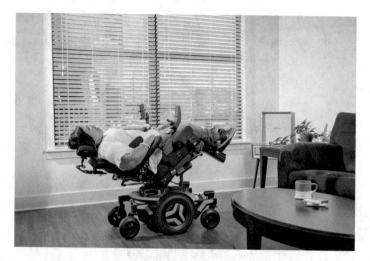

Fig. 2.10   Power tilt and recline; Permobil

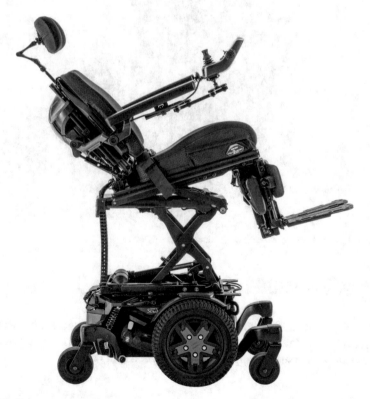

Fig. 2.11   Power seat elevation; Quantum Rehab

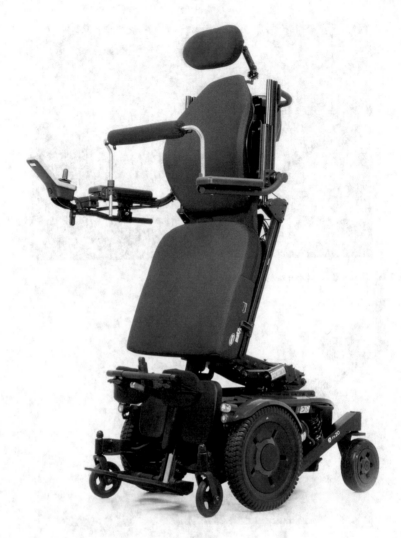

Fig. 2.12 Power standing wheelchair; Invacare

2.2.4   Seating System Considerations

Seating consists of various components. The primary components are the seat back and seat cushion. However, there are several other accessories that are essential for proper postural support and alignment and for good skin integrity.

2.2.4.1 Seat Cushions and Back Supports

Wheelchair seating consists of a back support and a seat cushion. Both components are essential for alignment, stability, and pressure relief. Poor seating can be detrimental to health, resulting in pressure injuries, pain, and deformity.

Back supports provide support to the spine and decrease stress into the spinal column. This in turn will allow for relaxation of the back muscles to maintain proper lumbar lordosis and a more upright posture, which improves comfort [18]. This support is found to be better than use of the fabric or upholstered backs that come standard with the wheelchair. Improved posture facilitates propulsion, functional task performance, and reach [19]. Persons with SCI should be seated with proper back support to encourage upper limb position, promote efficient propulsion, and facilitate function.

Back supports can vary in height and contour. The height should be tall enough to provide posterior support without interfering in function. Persons with lower-level SCI who self-propel a manual wheelchair require clearance of their scapula (also known as the shoulder blade) for efficient propulsion. Blocking the scapula interferes in full upper extremity range of motion, which in turn impacts efficiency of mobility. This requires a lower back support. Persons with higher-level SCI who utilize power wheelchairs for mobility require greater back support due to postural instability. A higher back is also necessary when using tilt and recline to ensure full posterior support when resting all the way back. Contour is dependent on asymmetrical postures and level of stability. The greater the instability, the deeper contour must be. Likewise, the greater the asymmetry, the deeper contour must be (Fig. 2.13).

Back supports play a role in skin integrity by encouraging improved overall alignment. When the spine is more neutral, the pelvis is more level, with decreased pressure into bony prominence.

Cushions are classified as general use, pressure relieving, positioning, and pressure relieving and positioning. General use cushions generally are a thinner foam and lack pressure relief capabilities. There are diagnostic requirements in order to qualify for a pressure relieving, positioning, or pressure relieving and positioning cushion under most insurances. Persons with SCI qualify for these and should be seated on a positioning and pressure relieving cushion at all times.

Wheelchair cushions are characterized as foam, air, and fluid. Foam cushions can come in a flat or contoured design. Air cushions generally consist of segmented air cells. Seat cushions play a large role in pressure relief due to the technology used. Research indicates that interface pressures are found to be higher in persons with less tissue. Persons with SCI are at greater risk for pressure injury due to less tissue under their bony prominence, including ischial tuberosities [20].

Pressure relief can occur in one of two forms: enveloping or orthotic offloading. Enveloping cushions allow for immersion of buttocks into the seat to increase contact area and decrease pressure. This is usually achieved most effectively with an air cushion (Fig. 2.14). Offloading cushions redistribute mass away from bony prominence and toward tissues that are better able to handle the load (Figs. 2.15 and 2.16). The decision for one design over another depends on the presence of pressure injury,

Fig. 2.13 Back supports;
Roho Agility Deep Back;
Permobil

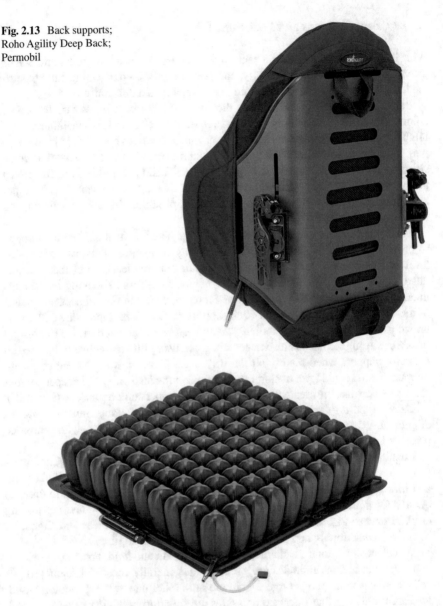

Fig. 2.14 Air cushion; Roho High Profile Quattro Select, Permobil

individual body shape, and risk of injury. The intention is to decrease risk of tissue deformation. When tissue deforms, there is a greater risk for the development of pressure injuries. While research has shown that in regard to pressure relief, air cell cushions generally result in less shear and provide optimal pressure relief, cushions that provide offloading provide the greatest pressure relief [21]. This is different from person to person, and as such each person with SCI should be assessed individually [22].

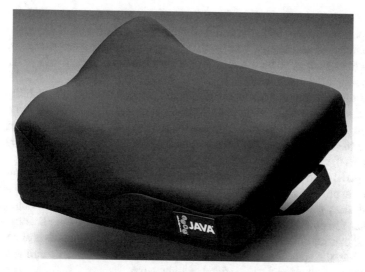

Fig. 2.15 Offloading cushion; Java Cushion, Ride Designs

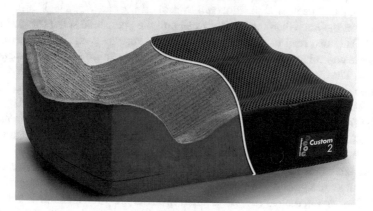

Fig. 2.16 Offloading cushion; Custom Ride Designs Cushion, Ride Designs

2.2.4.2   Positioning Accessory Components for Power Wheelchairs

There are several different mobility accessories that are essential for postural support and alignment. These include but are not limited to the following:

Lapbelt: A lapbelt is identified as a pelvic positioning device for use with the wheelchair. This stabilizes the pelvis back in the seat. This can benefit posture, skin integrity, and function. Padding is often used to allow for tightening up the belt without impacting the skin integrity of the pelvis during movements or when spasm is triggered. Lapbelts can also include four points of pull to better stabilize the pelvis when spasticity is stronger.

Headrest: The headrest provides posterior support to the head. Pads can be added on the side to support the head from flexing to one side or the other due to weakness, spasticity, or asymmetry. The headrest provides support when using power seat functions such as power tilt and recline, or when there is neck pain or fatigue, to allow for resting the head back.

Lateral trunk supports: Lateral trunk supports provide lateral trunk stability. These are often used with back supports with less contour. They can also allow for more customized placement of the lateral trunk support to support more extensive asymmetry and result in greater spinal control. They can be swung aside, removed, or are fixed to the back.

Pelvic pads: Also known as hip guides, these are mounted on the side of the wheelchair to provide a lateral block to the pelvis, so the pelvis does not shift out to the side. They provide stability and can control postural changes from both gravitational forces and spasticity. They are an important part of the seating system since control of the pelvis impacts spinal position. When the pelvis slides out to the side, the spine flexes to the side and results in worsening overall alignment. These are padded and can be fixed or removable.

Thigh supports: Lateral thigh supports provide distal support to the upper leg to maintain a more neutral position and control rolling out. When legs roll outward, wider at the knee than the hip, they can pull the pelvis and spine forward in the seat. This can lead to worsening asymmetry. Persons with SCI often lack the muscle control to maintain their legs in neutral and require an external support to do so. These can be of varying sizes and can be fixed or removable.

Gel supports: Gel can be placed on any support surface to decrease pressure, including headrests, armpads, footplates, pelvic pads, and thigh supports. These are used for persons who have pressure injuries or are at risk for pressure injuries at the elbows, back of the head, heels and balls of the feet, hips, and distal femur. This is only a partial list of placement of gel supports.

Joystick knobs for power wheelchairs: The standard joystick knob is a small knob that sticks straight up. For persons with higher-level SCI and impairment in prehension, an alternative support is often necessary. Options include a large ball, goal post, mushroom, and tall stick. There are several other off-the-shelf supports that exist, as well as the opportunity for customization.

2.2.5 *Insurance Considerations for Wheelchair Acquisition*

The wheelchairs mentioned above are considered complex rehabilitation technology (CRT). Because they are medical devices and are reimbursed through insurance, extensive documentation is required for authorization. The paperwork is usually generated by the therapist, in the form of the Letter of Medical Necessity, and signed off on by the physician. Often chart notes are also required, including special documentation called face to face notes. These documents, combined with pricing and prescriptions from the rehabilitation technology supplier, are gathered to form the packet submitted to insurance. Insurance reviews these documents and either approves, denies, or requests additional documentation. When denied, the person with SCI has the opportunity to appeal. The time frame can range from 2 to 6 months from evaluation to provision of the equipment.

Under the Medicare Local Coverage Determination (LCD), an ultralightweight K0005 wheelchair is only covered if the individual is a full-time wheelchair user and requires individualized custom fitting with accommodation to axle plate configuration, camber, and seat and back angles which are not possible with the K0001 through K0004. Furthermore, the individual must undergo a specialty evaluation by a licensed/certified medical professional (LCMP), such as an OT or PT, or physician who is trained not only in the assessment process but who also is capable of properly documenting the wheelchair and its features. Finally, the wheelchair must be provided by a Rehabilitative Technology Supplier (RTS) that employs a RESNA-certified Assistive Technology Professional (ATP) who specializes in wheelchairs. The ATP must have direct contact and involvement with the individual.

Most private insurances follow Medicare guidelines. Medicare is a federally funded program, administered by the federal government. This means that the guidelines are exactly the same from state to state. Private insurance plans are administered by the employer and are specific to the employer's plan. Medicaid is a federally funded program but is managed by each individual state. This means that guidelines can vary from state to state, and that what is reimbursed in one may not be reimbursed in another. In addition, many states have Medicaid plans that are managed by another company. While they still are managed by the state, there can be subtle variations between plans (i.e., some plans follow Medicare guidelines).

Medicare currently only reimburses equipment that is required full time for use in the home when completing mobility-related activities of daily living. If the equipment is not needed in the home, Medicare will not provide coverage for this device. Medicaid however provides coverage for community use. Sometimes, persons with SCI require a manual wheelchair full time in their home but a PAW in the community. If the person with SCI has Medicare (or a private insurance) and Medicaid, the wheelchair would be submitted to their primary plan, and the PAW request would be submitted to Medicaid.

2.2.6 Other Therapeutic Technologies and Interventions

There are several other technologies to consider when working with the person with SCI. Some are essential for function, while others are beneficial to rehabilitate the person with SCI both physically and emotionally.

2.2.6.1 Bathroom Equipment

Bathroom equipment consists of equipment for the toilet or the tub. The most basic toilet seat is a commode. This is a raised seat with an opening that can be placed over the toilet to facilitate completion of one's bowel and bladder regimen. There is the option for an opening for access. This can be in the front, side, or rear. It is important to know what location is easiest for access when the person with SCI is performing their routine and order a device that is properly configured for this. Toilet commodes can be statically placed over the toilet or can roll on wheels into the bathroom. This allows for a transfer to take place in the bedroom, for example, and then to move into the bathroom. The wheels can be small (attendant propelled) or larger (self-propelled). Larger wheels result in an increased overall width, which can interfere in doorway access. The seat can be hard plastic or padded. For persons with SCI, the padded option is preferred to decrease risk of pressure injury since completion of a bowel program can take some time.

For the tub the most basic model is the transfer tube bench, with two feet in the tub and two out. This allows for transfer onto the bench and then swinging one's legs into the tub. Another newer design is the sliding system, which consists of a commode that is pushed into the bathroom and attached to a track that is put in place in the tub, and then the seat is slid into the tub along the track. This decreases the need for transfers and can be a safer option for persons with increased spasticity or impaired skin integrity. Like the bath chair, tub systems can be hard plastic or padded. For persons with SCI, the padded option is preferred to decrease the risk of pressure injury.

2.2.6.2 Standing Frame

A standing frame is a device that stabilizes the person with SCI in a standing position. There are many benefits to standing, including range of motion, spasticity management, bone density, skin integrity, vital organ capacity, bowel and bladder function, and perceived self-image and self-esteem [23]. Persons with SCI identify increased bladder emptying and bowel management with regular standing programs. Static weight bearing results in a constant stretch into the joint, encouraging range of motion and decreasing severity of spasticity. Standing upright results in the pelvis tipping forward, removing all pressure from the seated surface and promoting good skin integrity. This position is also found to decrease long-term effects of back pain. Finally, standing brings the user into an upright position, which results in them being at a higher height and in turn improves self-image. The benefits of standing are strongly supported by the research [14]. For this reason, a standing frame should be incorporated into regular rehabilitation for persons with SCI.

2.2.6.3 Exoskeleton

Exoskeletons are classified as medical devices. The exoskeleton is a battery-powered robotic orthotic suit that enables standing and walking. The suit is placed over the persons limbs, providing powered movement at the hips and knees to initiate standing and walking. This can be used with persons with SCI with injuries at various spinal levels. It is a safe ambulation device with many health benefits [24]. This is newer technology that is not yet readily available or covered by insurance.

2.2.6.4 Electrical Stimulation

Dynamic electrical stimulation has been found to increase vascularization and muscle fiber area [25]. Electrical stimulation training consists of placement of electrodes at neuromuscular motor points in the legs, which fire alternatively. The person with SCI is seated in a cycle ergometer, with the legs moved automatically, while the motor points are stimulated.

2.2.6.5 Locomotive Training

Locomotive training involves suspension of the person with SCI in a harness over a treadmill (some systems can be used without treadmill and over a floor), with step training using body weight support. Therapists sit on either side of the person with SCI, moving the upper and lower extremities to simulate walking movements [26]. The goal is to use sensory information to stimulate spinal cord activity-dependent plasticity. There is some research that indicates that therapy that consists of repetition of task can retrain the nervous system to recover motor tasks [6].

2.2.6.6 Sports Devices

Sports wheelchairs are specifically designed for proper fit, minimal weight, and durability. The design of these wheelchairs is specific to the sport itself. Participation in sports has been found an effective tool to improve stamina and strength. It has also been found to increase community integration and improve perception of self and outlook on life after SCI. Sports wheelchairs are designed to create a close fit, like an orthotic device, so that the wheelchair is a continuation of the human body [27]. Camber is usually significantly larger in these devices as compared to one's day-to-day wheelchair. This is to create increased stability and responsiveness. In contact sports it also has the benefit of creating distance between the user and their opponent and to protect the user's hands. Again, the design is specific to the sport being played, which should be taken into consideration when pursuing a sports wheelchair.

Resources

- American Spinal Cord Injury Association
  asia-spinalinjury.org
- Model System Knowledge Center
  msktc.org
- United Spinal Association
  unitedspinal.org
- Christopher and Dana Reeve Foundation
  christopherreeve.org
- NCART: National Coalition for Assistive and Rehabilitation Technology
  ncart.us
- Access to CRT
  access2CRT.org
- ITEM Coalition: Independence Through Enhancement of Medicare and Medicaid
  itemcoalition.org
- NRRTS: National Registry of Rehabilitation Technology Suppliers
  nrrts.org
- LCD Manual and Power Wheelchairs
  cms.gov
- Clinician Task Force
  cliniciantaskforce.us
- ABLEDATA
  abledata.com
- Michael, E., Sytsma, T., & Cowan, R. E. (2020). A primary care provider's guide to wheelchair prescription for persons with spinal cord injury. *Topics in Spinal Cord Injury Rehabilitation, 26*(2), 100–107.

References

1. Chen, Y., DeVivo, M. J., Richards, J. S., & SanAgustin, T. B. (2016). Spinal cord injury model systems: Review of program and national database from 1970 to 2015. *Archives of Physical Medicine and Rehabilitation, 97*(10), 1797–1804.
2. Wang, T. Y., Park, C., Zhang, H., Rahimpour, S., Murphy, K. R., Goodwin, C. R., Karikari, I. O., Than, K. D., Shaffrey, C. I., Foster, N., & Abd-El-Barr, M. M. (2021). Management of acute traumatic spinal cord injury: A review of the literature. *Frontiers in Surgery, 8*, 698736.
3. Behrman, A. L., & Harkema, S. J. (2007). Physical rehabilitation as an agent for recovery after spinal cord injury. *Physical Medicine and Rehabilitation Clinics of North America, 18*(2), 183–202.
4. Waters, R. L., Adkins, R. H., Yakura, J. S., & Sie, I. (1994). Motor and sensory recovery following incomplete tetraplegia. *Archives of Physical Medicine and Rehabilitation, 75*(3), 306–311.
5. Angel, S., Kirkevold, M., & Pedersen, B. D. (2011). Rehabilitation after spinal cord injury and the influence of the professional's support (or lack thereof). *Journal of Clinical Nursing, 20*(11–12), 1713–1722.
6. Wolpaw, J. R., & Tennissen, A. M. (2001). Activity-dependent spinal cord plasticity in health and disease. *Annual Review of Neuroscience, 24*(1), 807–843.

7. Csikszentmihalyi, M. (1990). *Flow: The psychology of optimal experience*. HarperCollins.
8. Foy, T., Perritt, G., Thimmaiah, D., Heisler, L., Offutt, J. L., Cantoni, K., et al. (2011). Occupational therapy treatment time during inpatient spinal cord injury rehabilitation. *The Journal of Spinal Cord Medicine, 34*(2), 162–175.
9. National Spinal Cord Injury Statistical Center. (2017). *Facts and figures at a glance*. University of Alabama at Birmingham.
10. Cheng, C. L., Plashkes, T., Shen, T., Fallah, N., Humphreys, S., O'Connell, C., et al. (2017). Does specialized inpatient rehabilitation affect whether or not people with traumatic spinal cord injury return home? *Journal of Neurotrauma, 34*(20), 2867–2876.
11. Ditunno, P. L., Patrick, M., Stineman, M., & Ditunno, J. F. (2008). Who wants to walk? Preferences for recovery after SCI: A longitudinal and cross-sectional study. *Spinal Cord, 46*(7), 500–506.
12. Papadimitriou, C. (2008). Becoming en-wheeled: The situated accomplishment of re-embodiment as a wheelchair user after spinal cord injury. *Disability & Society, 23*(7), 691–704.
13. Paralyzed Veterans of America Consortium for Spinal Cord Medicine. (2005). Preservation of upper limb function following spinal cord injury: A clinical practice guideline for health-care professionals. *Journal of Spinal Cord Medicine, 28*(5), 434–470.
14. Dicianno, B. E., Morgan, A., Lieberman, J., & Rosen, L. (2013). *RESNA position on the application of wheelchair standing devices: 2013 current state of the literature*. Technical report, Rehabilitation Engineering and Assistive Technology.
15. Herberts, P., Kadefors, R., Hogfors, C., & Sigholm, G. (1984). Shoulder pain and heavy manual labor. *Clinical Orthopaedics & Related Research, 191*, 166–178.
16. Bjelle, A., Hagberg, M., & Michaelsson, G. (1979). Clinical and ergonomic factors in prolonged shoulder pain among industrial workers. *Scandinavian Journal of Work, Environment & Health, 5*(3), 205–210.
17. Wang, Y. T., Kim, C. K., Ford, H. T., III, & Ford, H. T., Jr. (1994). Reaction force and EMG analyses of wheelchair transfers. *Perceptual & Motor Skills, 79*, 763–766.
18. Makhsous, M., Lin, F., Hendrix, R. W., Hepler, M., & Zhang, L. Q. (2003). Sitting with adjustable ischial and back supports: Biomechanical changes. *Spine, 28*, 1113–1121, discussion 1121–1122.
19. Presperin Pedersen, J., Smith, C., Dahlin, M., Henry, M., Jones, J., McKenzie, K., Sevigny, M., & Yingling, L. (2022). Wheelchair backs that support the spinal curves: Assessing postural and functional changes. *The Journal of Spinal Cord Medicine, 45*(2), 194–203.
20. Brienza, D., Vallely, J., Karg, P., Akins, J., & Gefen, A. (2018). An MRI investigation of the effects of user anatomy and wheelchair cushion type on tissue deformation. *Journal of Tissue Viability, 27*(1), 42–53.
21. Damiao, J., & Gentry, T. (2021). A systematic review of the effectiveness of pressure relieving cushions in reducing pressure injury. *Assistive Technology*, 1–5. https://doi.org/10.1080/10400435.2021.2010148
22. Sonenblum, S. E., Ma, J., Sprigle, S. H., Hetzel, T. R., & Cathcart, J. M. (2018). Measuring the impact of cushion design on buttocks tissue deformation: An MRI approach. *Journal of Tissue Viability, 27*(3), 162–172.
23. Dunn, R. B., Walter, J. S., Lucero, Y., Weaver, F., Langbein, E., Fehr, L., et al. (1998). Follow-up assessment of standing mobility device users. *Assistive Technology, 10*(2), 84–93.
24. Miller, L. E., Zimmermann, A. K., & Herbert, W. G. (2016). Clinical effectiveness and safety of powered exoskeleton-assisted walking in patients with spinal cord injury: Systematic review with meta-analysis. *Medical Devices (Auckland, NZ), 9*, 455.
25. Crameri, R. M., Cooper, P., Sinclair, P. J., Bryant, G., & Weston, A. (2004). Effect of load during electrical stimulation training in spinal cord injury. *Muscle & Nerve: Official Journal of the American Association of Electrodiagnostic Medicine, 29*(1), 104–111.
26. Sisto, S. A., Forrest, G. F., & Faghri, P. D. (2008). Technology for mobility and quality of life in spinal cord injury [analyzing a series of options available]. *IEEE Engineering in Medicine and Biology Magazine, 27*(2), 56–68.
27. Cooper, R. A., & De Luigi, A. J. (2014). Adaptive sports technology and biomechanics: Wheelchairs. *PM&R, 6*(8), S31–S39.

Chapter 3
Subjective Experience

In Chap. 1, the physical effects of spinal cord injury (SCI) were presented, including the immediate direct effects on the body and the secondary complications. These effects are often easier to comprehend as they are visible. One can see the change in the physical body. Though they may not understand the outcome, they are aware of the modification based upon the visual tangible change. This chapter examines the qualitative components of SCI. It focuses on quality of life and life satisfaction, delving into each change and how it affects the psyche of the person with SCI. While each person with SCI experiences their changed body differently, there are similarities occurring among all persons with SCI.

3.1 The Subjective Meaning of SCI

Life satisfaction and quality of life (QOL) are two different concepts. One's perception of one's quality of life is the differential between their internal self-appraisal and the external appraisal of others [1]. It is the differential between how they see themselves and how they perceive they are seen by others. QOL is a measurement of overall well-being. Life satisfaction is a component of QOL. Both play a significant role in subjective experience.

Research reveals that life satisfaction among most persons with SCI improves over time, from 6 months post-injury to between 1 and 5 years after discharge from rehabilitation [2–4]. The factors that affect a positive outcome are age, time since onset of injury, education level, being in a solid relationship, lower level of injury, and incomplete injury [2]; functional independence [3, 4]; less pain [3–6]; and increased mobility [7–9].

Regardless of level of injury, both QOL and life satisfaction are directly impacted by the diagnosis of SCI and secondary complications related to SCI [7, 10, 11]. In reality, every component of life is impacted by the onset of SCI. The change in the

© The Author(s) 2022
J. Lieberman, *The Physical, Personal, and Social Impact of Spinal Cord Injury*,
SpringerBriefs in Public Health, https://doi.org/10.1007/978-3-031-18652-3_3

physical body and in physical ability directly influences QOL and life satisfaction. Changes in physical capabilities result not only in changes in the ability to complete daily functional activities but also in how one perceives one's social role [12]. This change in ability, social role, and self-perception all plays a role in satisfaction with life.

The World Health Organization has organized the consequences of disease into three classifications: impairment, disability, and handicap [13]. The impairment is the SCI. The disability is the restriction created by the impairment, which for the person with SCI is loss of motor and/or sensory function. The handicap is the environmental factor that interferes in normal life. The environment handicaps the person with SCI due to the need to use a wheelchair in a predominantly inaccessible world. This is not an internal factor but rather environmental.

Those with greater handicap report decreased satisfaction with life. The handicap is identified as the result of the impairment, or disability, that prevents those skills needed to fulfill one's role, including mobility, social support, environmental access, and occupational role [9].

Life satisfaction is a deeply personal concept. Each person with SCI perceives their satisfaction with life differently. There are however factors that play a strong role in the overall perception of life satisfaction, including societal and cultural influences. One's satisfaction with life is correlated with the comparison of their personal circumstances and their perception of what is normal. One's perception of what is normal comes from their interactions with others. One's sense of self is therefore maintained via their interactions with others [14]. As the person with SCI experiences an alteration in their interactions with others due to physical, emotional, social, and environmental changes, their perception of what is normal changes, and their satisfaction with life decreases. However, over time, these perceptions are frequently found to reverse themselves.

Because this is a deeply personal concept, the only relevant assessment of life satisfaction and quality of life for the person with SCI is their own well-being. For this reason, onset of SCI does not have to diminish quality of life at all. For some, it can actually improve quality of life [15]. If the proper resources are available, including social support, rehabilitation, and assistance with coping, and if the environmental and social factors do not interfere in engagement, the quality of life for the person with SCI does not have to diminish.

Knowledge that engagement and participation in life are predictors of overall well-being reinforces the importance of rehabilitation programs. The goal of rehabilitation is to promote function and reduce disability. Through engaging with clinical staff and other persons with disabilities, opportunities for successful mobility and community participation increase [16]. This can lead to improved quality of life and well-being, which is essential for achieving a life worth living. Therefore, it becomes paramount that the person with SCI participates in rehabilitation as soon after injury as possible, in a setting that is experienced with working with persons with SCI (i.e., SCIMS).

3.2 Loneliness

Relationships are essential for health and well-being. People who do not have strong social relationships are found to have poorer physical and mental health outcomes [17]. A lack of relationships often leads to social isolation, which can lead to increased feelings of loneliness. This experience is however personal, supporting the idea that quality relationships are more important than quantity.

Persons with SCI identify experiencing higher levels of loneliness than the general population. Several factors impact this, including environmental, social, and physical. This is an important experience to identify due to the correlations between loneliness with depression and depression with health.

The disconnection that occurs for a person after a trauma like SCI is body, mind, and soul. It occurs simultaneously between the body and society. One can think of the severing of the spinal cord like the severing of normalcy or what is perceived as being normal. The person with SCI begins to view themselves as they would have viewed others with SCI: as victims or abnormal [18]. Our preconceived concepts of normalcy create a sense of being abnormal.

This is present in all facets of life, including medical and rehabilitation settings. The person with SCI exists in a special world compared to those treating them, so that sense of different is ingrained. In essence, healthcare unintentionally reinforces the concept of abnormal [19]. While the goal of the treatment team is to rehabilitate the person with SCI and to promote functional independence, the staff are subconsciously aware of disability by the pure nature of knowing they are working with persons with SCI. The treatment team specialized in working with persons with SCI are often more acutely aware of the possible positive outcomes during rehabilitation. They are however also aware of what the person with SCI may no longer be able to do, and that concept remains an unintentional thought of the members of the treatment team during intervention.

The cultural fabrication of disability creates the belief that those who are different are not normal. Social and environmental barriers reinforce this by denying access of the person in a wheelchair to certain environments. The person with SCI becomes a stranger to themselves upon awakening not just because their sense of who they were in the world was altered due to neural damage but also because they must now experience their lives as outsiders in an able-bodied world. Prior to injury, there was no need to think about obstacles. Everyone just went about their business. Now, every aspect of every activity needs to be conceptualized to promote participation.

Because disability is stigmatized, it is hard to think of oneself as normal after SCI. The ability to internalize being still "normal" becomes essential for recovery. This however is not easy since we are predisposed to believing that impairment is not normal [20]. The desire to regain a sense of self as normal requires internalizing that people with disabilities are still normal, and to not perceive the disability as a stigma [21]. This is important, because until the individual develops a sense of normalcy, they will retain a feeling of being disabled.

There are ways however to create this sense of normalcy. For example, planning becomes a key component to integration. Having knowledge of locations and environments that will be accessed allows for planning specific functions, such as management of bladder, avoidance of barriers, and access to locations. Planning in effect creates normalcy because if performed covertly, others are unaware [21]. Planning allows for controlling the situation and being the instigator of change, which can result in a feeling of perceived independence.

Participation in leisure activities can also decrease severity of loneliness. There is a correlation between participation in leisure activities and loneliness, which goes both ways. Persons who are lonely participate less in leisure activities, while simultaneously persons who participate in fewer leisure activities identify increased feelings of loneliness [22]. Increased participation for the person with SCI leads to increased engagement with one's environment and with society. Feelings of loneliness become less intense the greater the frequency of participation. For the person with SCI, participating in support groups, peer groups, and life challenging activities becomes an important component to help control feelings of loneliness and isolation.

3.3   The Overarching Concept of Time

The person with SCI is a constant memorial to time. The moment of trauma to the spine splits the past from the present and alters the future. All persons have a concept of their lived life and the expectation of what the future will be. the future being tomorrow, next week, next year. Then the SCI occurs, and everything the person with SCI believed they were and were going to become is taken away. People measure time as a continuum from past to present to future. This is a circuitous pattern. Reflection on life occurs in the moment, with fluctuations between memories of the past and thoughts of the future. When there is an event as traumatic as a SCI, there is a disruption of this pattern. Because there is no past experience with SCI to relate to, the future becomes unclear. This leads to the inability to conceive of a meaningful future. For the person with SCI, time stops because of the disruption to life expectations based upon their previous goals. However, these goals can change. The ideas of the past may previously have been school years, whereas now they can be the previous weeks or months before when movement was not possible.

This is important to understand when supporting the person with SCI, whether as family, friend, or healthcare provider. As the person with SCI tries to move through their day, their concept of the present and future is dependent on their past experiences and future hopes. Memories of the past and thoughts of oneself in the future create meaning for the present. For example, drawing awareness to the past week when the person could not raise their arm to the present when they can feed themselves changes their perception of the future from being unable to capable. Acknowledgement of small goals can positively alter thoughts of the future.

Wheelchair use is a constant reminder of the past. For the person with SCI, using a wheelchair is necessary. As the person with SCI sits in and uses the wheelchair, they are reminded that they once walked. The present is filled with memories of the past. There is no way to avoid this way of thinking. The idea of no longer being able to perform activities that were once so meaningful results in increased distress, especially if those activities form the foundation of one's identity. However, the SCI introduces new identities due to a change in embodiment and restructuring of consciousness. The disruption in life's expectations creates the chance to remake oneself. For some individuals with SCI, this actually creates an opportunity to start over, to experience a new present and possible future. In essence, a "clean slate" for a new life [23–25]. Some persons with SCI identify the date of their injury as their second birthday. They see this new future as a rebirth.

3.4 Initial Reactions to a Changed Body

Our body is our expression of the world [26]. SCI results in changes to how the person with SCI experiences their environment and their body in the environment. The trauma results in the concrete severing of communication below the location of injury. This damage is not only to the nerves that are responsible for sensation but also to those nerves that are responsible for muscle mobility. The damage is also to the identity of the person with SCI. If one's sense of one's self as a being in the world is rooted in the mind-body connection [27], then it seems awareness of oneself at one's core will be altered when sensorimotor alteration occurs.

The body's sense of self comes from the integration of sensory feedback and motor responses. After SCI this is disrupted, disrupting the sense of self. This can lead to feelings of being a foreigner in a body that was once so familiar. Some describe a SCI as a disease of consciousness due to the loss of connection between mind and body [28]. Because of the lost sense of self in space, there is a loss of sense of identity in the world. After the initial injury, many persons with SCI identify an awareness that something is terribly wrong due to the inability to move. This difficulty with understanding the inability to move is often due to rote memories of moving in space.

The sudden disconnect that occurs at the time of injury is a fracture in one's relationship with the physical world. Some persons with SCI identify feeling like a foreigner in a body that had once been so familiar with no awareness of what happened. Robert Murphy (1987) identified that sudden paralysis can trigger the process of separation from one's body and one's self [29]. There is a lost sense of self because of no true awareness of one's body being in the world. This is most apparent immediately after the injury and during the initial hospitalization and rehabilitation phase.

It is important to understand the perception of the disruption of one's sense of body. Considerations should be made by the treatment team to the reaction of the person with SCI to medical events that occur during hospitalization and rehabilitation. For example, the onset of orthostatic hypotension is terrifying. The negative effects of gravity when brought up to sit, can result in the spontaneous fear of loss of control of the new body. The loss of muscle control results in the loss of structural support of the body. Not only is the person with SCI unable to hold themselves up against gravity, but the loss of muscle control results in the rush of blood to their lower body when transitioning from lying to sitting and sitting to standing. As the blood pools in their lower body, there are often moments of loss of consciousness. This is humbling and scary. Furthermore, staffing often doesn't effectively prepare the person with SCI for this event to occur, and they do not always anticipate this response. Communication becomes essential and is a large aspect of education. It becomes extremely important, for example, to explain what is occurring to the body during changes in position. It helps the persons with SCI to understand the changes to their body and empowers them to develop their voice when experiencing certain symptoms. Communication allows for dignity and respect.

Another consideration is the experience of having a pressure injury. The obvious alteration of the body is unsettling. As explored earlier, pressure injuries result when blood flow is blocked to tissues and they die. The damage can be deep through the skin, muscle, and down to the bone. It is important to consider not just the damage to the body but how it is perceived. The awareness of the sense of deformity, whether through smell or pain, is terrifying. A pressure injury is deeply embedded in each person's experience and their changed body image [30]. It can be shocking for the person with SCI that they have developed something that is so horribly disfiguring, especially when they cannot feel the pressure injury. It is a reminder of the disruption that has occurred to their body and how much they can no longer control.

SCI directly impacts one's quality of life by altering one's perception of one's health, independence, hope for emotional and sexual relationships with others, having a family, and the future possibility of being employed. Bladder management and the avoidance of urinary accidents are a primary factor in the interruption of achieving this quality of life [31]. Persons with SCI cannot control their bowel or bladder systems and are at high risk of accident during the day. This can lead to decreased participation in daily activities in the community due to anxiety over having an accident and the fear of experiencing embarrassment. However, a regular bowel and bladder program can significantly decrease the incidence of accident and in turn help improve quality of life.

Sexuality plays a critical role in coping with one's disability and in self-esteem. Due to physical changes after sustaining a SCI, physical adaptations are required in order to achieve sexual adjustment after SCI. The concept as a sexual being for the person with SCI must be redefined. Society views sexuality as a privilege of the able-bodied [32]. Sex has historically been connected with the ideas of reproduction, and society views persons with disabilities as not proper candidates to reproduce [33]. For the person with SCI, the body doesn't move or feel the same due to the changes the body has experienced. Conceptually, the body cannot engage as it previously had. Pre-injury perceptions of normal sexual relations and sex acts interfere in their belief of sexuality. The person believes they are no longer normal and therefore can no longer have a normal sexual relationship. These ideals of normalcy are based on previous experiences and instilled societal norms of what sex should be like. Society says that sexuality is a product of performance and genital function. For the person with SCI, both are altered. Their performance is different due to the changed body, and there are changes in sensation and function of the sex organs. These societal notions combined with the changed body lead to feelings of inadequacy and inability. The person with SCI loses hope [33].

Sex and sexual pleasure connect people. It can help decrease one's sense of isolation and loneliness and increase integration into society. The person with SCI is already struggling with feelings of low self-esteem and isolation. The changed body no longer being able to engage in sex "normally" magnifies these emotions. In order to decrease the negative effects on perceptions of sexuality and pleasure, it is important to educate the person with SCI shortly after their injury ways to relearn how to experience pleasure. This becomes essential not only for sexual pleasure but also for self-esteem and to decrease feelings of loneliness. While these conversations need to be initiated by healthcare providers, research has identified that persons with SCI feel more comfortable discussing sex and sexuality with other persons with SCI [34].

All persons bring a preconceived notion of sex and sexuality to the table. It becomes essential to understand how the person with SCI perceives sex and what their sexual issues are due to the onset of SCI. A thorough history of diagnoses and medications will provide information on metabolic and neurotropic factors impacting the body. Providing the person with SCI with education on all the factors involved and techniques on relearning arousal and sexuality can positively impact self-esteem and overall satisfaction with life.

The rehabilitation team can play a huge role in recovery of sexuality and sexual identity [34]. While addressing sexuality in a team approach with multiple team members involved, it is often the role of the nurse and the OT to address this. Sex is an activity of daily living, which is the OT area of specialty. The nurse provides a safe space in which the person with SCI can explore and be respected. However, education should not end upon discharge. Discharge into the community is when the person with SCI comes to terms with their capabilities in the real world.

3.5 Subjective Experience of Wheelchair Use

The wheelchair is the extension of the user's body [35]. It is necessary for the person with SCI to engage in activities. The wheelchair allows the person with SCI to live independently and successfully in their environment. Participation is an essential component to quality of life. The wheelchair makes participation possible.

Mobility has always been equated with freedom and choice [36]. For the able-bodied population, the ability to freely move in one's home and community, managing environmental barriers and obstacles, increases opportunity and choice, which in turn increases level of independence. For this reason, wheelchair use has historically been viewed by society with prejudice [37, 38]. This has influenced how persons with disabilities view themselves and how they are viewed and treated by others.

These preconceived notions of wheelchair use impact how persons with SCI are treated in the world. Creating a world full of environmental obstacles, including stairs, inaccessible public spaces, restaurants, bathrooms, and transportation, reinforces the demoralization of persons with SCI who rely on wheelchairs. By preventing access to environments, they are prevented from engaging with those who do not require wheelchairs for mobility. Again, this reinforces the "them versus us" mentality.

Social isolation occurs because of wheelchair use in a world full of structural and social barriers. This directly impacts meaningful existence for people with SCI and creates a loss of identity [29]. Aside from the personal experience with the physical change that occurs, use of a wheelchair is felt as demoralizing. Sitting in a wheelchair is felt as demoralizing not only because of the awareness of no longer being able-bodied but also because of the loss of stature due to being lower to the ground [39, 40].

There are several themes around wheelchair use and the perception of being disabled [41]. These are humiliation, frustration, loss, and humility. The wheelchair is viewed as socially demeaning and defines the user. However, many persons with SCI also perceive the wheelchair as being an extension of themselves and a vehicle of freedom [27]. In essence, the wheelchair is viewed as both enabling and disabling.

Persons with SCI identify the wheelchair as the greatest barrier in participation [35]. The impairment is not the limiting factor, but rather the equipment needed to manage the impairment is what handicaps the individual. Access can either promote or impede participation. Doorway widths, curbs, and steps hills are all environmental factors that impact performance based upon how the wheelchair can maneuver them. The weight, size, and maneuverability of the wheelchair all play a role in how the person with SCI maneuvers in their interior and exterior environments. The fit is also important in participation. A poorly fitted wheelchair results in discomfort, imbalance, and decreased function. These factors limit participation [42]. Since participation in life is correlated to well-being, it makes sense that the wheelchair is viewed by the person with SCI as playing a major role in their quality of life.

There are both objective and subjective experiences in this world. For the person with SCI, how they perceive their world is influenced not just by their injury but also on how they experience their injury while using a wheelchair. The SCI can cause neurological, medical, and orthopedic symptoms. So can wheelchair use, with upper limb pain from repetitive use, spinal asymmetry from the effect of gravity on absent musculature, and pressure injury from sitting in the wheelchair all day long. For this reason, exploration of wheelchair use with the person with SCI is just as important as educating them on all the consequences of their SCI. All these factors influence how the person with SCI senses and experiences their world.

3.6   Grief and Depression

Experiences of grief and depression are prevalent after SCI. This is a result of the loss of the previous identity with no ability to conceive of a meaningful future. Each reaction is different and as such should be addressed differently because not all reactions can be treated the same.

Grief is a response to loss. It represents several different reactions, including yearning, avoiding, and having difficulty accepting what was lost, as well as being confused about one's role in life. It presents itself as sadness, anger, guilt, anxiety, hopelessness, and despair [43]. In most people, this reaction is short lived, but in some it can persist beyond 6 months. Grief and depression are two very distinct reactions after SCI [44]. The grief experienced after SCI is related to either loss or traumatic distress (shock). The loss is the feelings of emptiness and confusion that part of the person had died or that life was meaningless. The grief reaction is different from all other reactions, including other grief reactions. For the person with SCI, the grief reaction is traumatic in nature. Neuropsychological intervention around grief often includes reassurances of one's circumstances. But for the person with SCI, sometimes reassuring them of their circumstances and capabilities can be acutely more detrimental. There are newer therapies geared to treating grief that are a combination of cognitive behavioral and interpersonal techniques. For this reason, it is important that the person with SCI is properly assessed for their response to sudden traumatic disability in order to guide them in the best way to achieve a sense of a meaningful life.

If, on the other hand, the person is identified to be experiencing major depressive disorder, introduction of psychotherapy and pharmacological medications early on is often of great benefit. Depression can occur at any time in the life of the person with SCI and is found to be highest within the first few years; however, it is known to improve over time [45]. Untreated depression after sustaining SCI can lead to poor outcomes in both short-term and long-term rehabilitation (Judd, 1986). Rates of depression can be as high as 20%, with 15% of those who are depressed experiencing suicidal ideation.

Suicide is three times higher in the spinal cord-injured population compared to the general population [46]. Some people identify the desire to die at different points of their life after sustaining their spinal cord injuries, with the highest rates of suicide occurring within the first 12 months [45]. These feelings are strongest as they are trying to re-habilitate and learn how to use their bodies.

While trying to regain mobility and perform day to day activities, there is daily awareness that the person with SCI is forever altered as they struggle to move. The inability to walk and the possibility of never walking again are hard to process. The knowledge that they would have to rely on a wheelchair for mobility for the reminder of their lives starts to sink in. The awareness of what the body cannot do is overwhelming, as every attempt at normal body movement fails.

Rehabilitation can decrease the severity of loss. Repetition and engagement can lead to small daily gains, which can lead to hope. For this reason, it is essential that the person with SCI continue to engage in active therapy even after discharge from the rehabilitation unit.

3.7   Hope

Hope is an essential component to recovery because it relieves debilitating suffering [47]. It is hard for the person with SCI to move forward from the traumatic disconnections they experience between mind and body. However, once the person with SCI is able to perceive of a future with their changed body, they can move forward with a new sense of identity. Re-evaluating what has occurred allows for conceptualizing a future which leads to hope. Hope can allow the person with SCI to look forward. It does not eliminate awareness of suffering and pain, but it does allow the person with SCI to see that they have a choice to realize their possibilities [48].

An important component of hope for the person with SCI is understanding who they were prior to their SCI. Developing an awareness that their exterior may have changed but their core remains the same can aid in establishing a sense of a life worth living. While most persons with SCI never imagine experiencing a change to their way of being in the world, they often ultimately decide that rather than giving up, they could live with this change [49].

Life for all persons, whether with or without SCI, is a continuous alteration in what is normal and what is not. Through daily performance of activities, we all fluctuate between feeling success and failure. But over time, it is possible to develop a sense of self and a feeling that life can be meaningful and worth living. It can take time, between 2 and 7 years, for a person with SCI to adjust to disability [15]. This adjustment occurs when the disability is no longer the primary concern in the life of the person with SCI.

While support from clinicians, friends, and family can assist in this process, it is one the person with SCI achieves on their own. There are factors that can aid in achieving this success. These include mentors and participation in community-based activities. Since our perception of normal is developed through our awareness of others, achieving success in the community around others who we perceive to be normal can lead to success and a sense of hope for the future.

3.8   Finding Meaning in Membership

Persons with SCI are different. Being different alienates persons with disabilities. For the person with SCI, their disability is felt as a "social malady" [29, p. 4]. Social and environmental barriers create the disability, not the individual. Meaningful relationships can be the bridge to "normal" society. They provide a valuable lens for seeing and believing in a future that they could not have imagined previously.

These relationships can be friends and family, spiritual relationships, and relationships with others with disabilities. These relationships are also temporal. They change over time, with different relationships taking precedent over others. At one point in time, encouragement by family and friends is necessary to move forward. At another point in time, one's faith becomes an avenue for keeping existential hope. And then at another point, relationships with others with disabilities in the form of peer mentors are the most important. It is important to understand this and offer these relationship opportunities so the person with SCI can find what is meaningful and necessary at any time.

Social supports found in familial and friend relationships have been found to play a very large role in well-being after SCI by decreasing grief/hopelessness and depression. However, it is not the quantity of support, but rather the quality [45]. Having a large support network does not decrease symptoms of depression and hopelessness. What has the greatest impact is the nature of these relationships and their quality. A strong social network creates a positive environment where one can engage with less stress. This benefits the person with SCI to achieve greater success through trial and error in a safer space.

Social support for persons with SCI in the form of close friendships can decrease severity of depression. It also leads to greater rates of satisfaction and physical function with increased social participation. While some statistics show that people with SCI are often single and have higher rates of divorce than the general population, there is a strong correlation between spousal support and QOL and well-being [50].

Spirituality has been found as a common theme among persons with SCI when attempting to recover from a traumatic event [51]. One's spirituality provides structure to understanding a more global meaning of SCI [49]. Belief in a higher power impacts how one deals with traumatic life events, such as SCI. For some persons with SCI, their existential hope leads to the belief that their survival after a traumatic SCI was either directly due to God or that their beliefs ultimately brought them a sense of peace living their life with a spinal cord injury [47]. Resilience has been found to originate from a belief in God and God's will, which is often associated with a positive outcome when recovering from an event like SCI. For persons with SCI, spirituality cannot only positively impact QOL, but it can also decrease incidence of depression [52]. Believing in a higher power provides the opportunity for finding meaning in one's life. For the person with SCI who is grappling with loss of body and sense of self, this is important for a meaningful recovery.

Relationships with persons with SCI can take on the form of peer mentorship. Peer mentorship is one of the strongest factors in development of an understanding of what is possible after SCI due to the experience of the peer mentor having lived with SCI. The peer's personal experiences and interactions normalize specific experiences the newly injured person is going through [53]. Hope becomes possible when informational and emotional support is provided by the peer with SCI to the newly injured person with SCI. They provide a glimpse of what is possible when the newly injured person is experiencing the unknown.

Peer mentors with SCI are individuals who have experienced SCI, and due to their unique life experience, they are best able to provide emotional, educational, motivational, and physical support. Peer mentors can provide persons with SCI with a realistic expectation of life with a spinal cord injury and show them how to engage with the community and others. This can promote adjustment and the willingness for increased community engagement [54]. This is achieved by providing both informational and emotional support. Informational support consists of information and advice. The peer with SCI can help problem solve ideas based upon their personal experience and provide education and information based upon their personal knowledge. Emotional support consists of empathy, understanding, and recognition of need. The peer with SCI has already experienced being newly injured in the social world of those without SCI. They have personal understanding of being paralyzed in an able-bodied world and the cultural ideals around disability. This unique experience makes the peer with SCI the ideal person to aid the person with SCI in reframing their own concept of disability [55].

Exposure to peer mentors early on after SCI has been found to result in increased self-efficacy and decreased incidence of rehospitalization [56]. Peer mentors provide a unique set of knowledge due to experience, and they can impart education on the skills needed for self-care. Acute rehabilitation stays have shortened over time. Persons with SCI are being discharged home with little knowledge over expectations due to feeling overwhelmed by their circumstances. This has led to an increase in hospitalization. Learning how to manage the health of their new body is challenging for the person with SCI. This leads to increased illness and infection. Peer mentors can educate the person with SCI on their personal experience with managing these new health challenges to decrease risk of rehospitalization.

Interaction with peer mentors has also been found to increase participation in community reintegration and employment and to improve life satisfaction. Due to the multitude of positive outcomes related to peer mentorship, rehabilitation-accrediting agencies now require proof of peer support in spinal cord and brain injury programs. However, there is not much consistency from program to program. If the acute rehabilitation setting lacks formal peer support, the person with SCI can contact local spinal cord injury organizations and chapters.

Resources
- Adjusting to Life After Spinal Cord Injury
  Model System Knowledge Center
  msktc.org
- United Spinal Association
  unitedspinal.org
- For Families Facing Spinal Cord Injuries
  FacingDisability.com
- Christopher and Dana Reeve Foundation
  christopherreeve.org

References

1. van Dijk, A. J. (2000). Quality of life assessment: Its integration in rehabilitation care through a model of daily living. *Scandinavian Journal of Rehabilitation Medicine, 32*(3), 104–110.
2. Shin, J. C., Goo, H. R., Yu, S. J., Kim, D. H., & Yoon, S. Y. (2012). Depression and quality of life in patients within the first 6 months after the spinal cord injury. *Annals of Rehabilitation Medicine, 36*(1), 119–125.
3. van Koppenhagen, C. F., Post, M. W., van der Woude, L. H., de Groot, S., de Witte, L. P., van Asbeck, F. W., et al. (2009). Recovery of life satisfaction in persons with spinal cord injury during inpatient rehabilitation. *American Journal of Physical Medicine & Rehabilitation, 88*(11), 887–895.
4. van Leeuwen, C. M., Post, M. W., Westers, P., van der Woude, L. H., de Groot, S., Sluis, T., & Lindeman, E. (2012). Relationships between activities, participation, personal factors, mental health, and life satisfaction in persons with spinal cord injury. *Archives of Physical Medicine and Rehabilitation, 93*(1), 82–89.
5. Kemp, B. J., & Krause, J. S. (1999). Depression and life satisfaction among people ageing with post-polio and spinal cord injury. *Disability & Rehabilitation, 21*(5–6), 241–249.
6. Westgren, N., & Levi, R. (1998). Quality of life and traumatic spinal cord injury. *Archives of Physical Medicine and Rehabilitation, 79*(11), 1433–1439.
7. Dijkers, M. P. J. M. (1999). Correlates of life satisfaction among persons with spinal cord injury. *Archives of Physical Medicine and Rehabilitation, 80*(8), 867–876.
8. Fuhrer, M. J., Rintala, D. H., Hart, K. A., Clearman, R., & Young, M. E. (1992). Relationship of life satisfaction to impairment, disability, and handicap among persons with spinal cord injury living in the community. *Archives of Physical Medicine and Rehabilitation, 73*(6), 552–557.
9. Putzke, J. D., Richards, J. S., Hicken, B. L., & DeVivo, M. J. (2002). Interference due to pain following spinal cord injury: Important predictors and impact on quality of life. *Pain, 100*(3), 231–242.
10. Buning, M. E., Angelo, J. A., & Schmeler, M. R. (2001). Occupational performance and the transition to powered mobility: A pilot study. *American Journal of Occupational Therapy, 55*(3), 339–344.
11. van Leeuwen, C. M., Post, M. W., Hoekstra, T., van der Woude, L. H., de Groot, S., Snoek, G. J., & Lindeman, E. (2011). Trajectories in the course of life satisfaction after spinal cord injury: Identification and predictors. *Archives of Physical Medicine and Rehabilitation, 92*(2), 207–213.
12. Hicken, B. L., Putzke, J. D., Novack, T., Sherer, M., & Richards, J. S. (2002). Life satisfaction following spinal cord and traumatic brain injury: A comparative study. *Journal of Rehabilitation Research and Development, 39*(3), 359–366.
13. World Health Organization. (1980). International classification of impairments, disabilities, and handicaps: A manual of classification relating to the consequences of disease, published in accordance with resolution WHA29. 35 of the twenty-ninth world health assembly, May 1976. World Health Organization.
14. Cantril, H. (1966). *The pattern of human concerns.* Rutgers University Press.
15. Dijkers, M. (1997). Quality of life after spinal cord injury: A meta analysis of the effects of disablement components. *Spinal Cord, 35*(12), 829.
16. Post, M., & Noreau, L. (2005). Quality of life after spinal cord injury. *Journal of Neurologic Physical Therapy, 29*(3), 139–146.
17. Hitzig, S. L., Cimino, S. R., Alavinia, M., Bassett-Gunter, R. L., Craven, B. C., & Guilcher, S. J. (2021). Examination of the relationships among social networks and loneliness on health and life satisfaction in people with spinal cord injury/dysfunction. *Archives of Physical Medicine and Rehabilitation, 102*(11), 2109–2116.
18. Papadimitriou, C. (2001). From dis-ability to difference: Conceptual and methodological issues in the study of physical disability. In S. K. Toombs (Ed.), *Handbook of phenomenology and medicine* (pp. 475–492). Kluwer.

19. Deegan, P. E. (1988). Recovery: The lived experience of rehabilitation. *Psychosocial Rehabilitation Journal, 11*(4), 11.
20. Papadimitriou, C. (2008b). The 'I' of the beholder: Phenomenological seeing in disability research. *Sports, Ethics and Philosophy, 2*(2), 216–233.
21. Suarez, N. C., Levi, R., & Bullington, J. (2013). Regaining health and wellbeing after traumatic spinal cord injury. *Journal of Rehabilitation Medicine, 45*(10), 1023–1027.
22. Santino, N., Larocca, V., Hitzig, S. L., Guilcher, S. J., Craven, B. C., & Bassett-Gunter, R. L. (2022). Physical activity and life satisfaction among individuals with spinal cord injury: Exploring loneliness as a possible mediator. *The Journal of Spinal Cord Medicine, 45*(2), 173–179.
23. Galli, G., & Pazzaglia, M. (2015). Commentary on: "The body social: an enactive approach to the self." A tool for merging bodily and social self in immobile individuals. *Frontiers in Psychology, 6*, 1–3.
24. Papadimitriou, C., & Stone, D. A. (2011). Addressing existential disruption in traumatic spinal cord injury: A new approach to human temporality in inpatient rehabilitation. *Disability and Rehabilitation, 33*(21–22), 2121–2133.
25. Seymour, W. (2002). Time and the body: Re-embodying time in disability. *Journal of Occupational Science, 9*(3), 135–142.
26. Merleau-Ponty, M. (2002). *Phenomenology of perception*. Routledge Classics.
27. Papadimitriou, C. (2008). Becoming en-wheeled: The situated accomplishment of re-embodiment as a wheelchair user after spinal cord injury. *Disability & Society, 23*(7), 691–704.
28. Cole, J. (2009). Impaired embodiment and intersubjectivity. *Phenomenology and the Cognitive Sciences, 8*(3), 343–360.
29. Murphy, R. (1990). *The silent body*. W.W. Norton.
30. Langemo, D. K., Melland, H., Hanson, D., Olson, B., & Hunter, S. (2000). The lived experience of having a pressure ulcer: A qualitative analysis. *Advances in Skin & Wound Care, 13*(5), 225–235.
31. Brillhart, B. (2004). Studying the quality of life and life satisfaction among persons with spinal cord injury undergoing urinary management. *Rehabilitation Nursing, 29*(4), 122–126.
32. Ricciardi, R., Szabo, C. M., & Poullos, A. Y. (2007). Sexuality and spinal cord injury. *Nursing Clinics of North America, 42*(4), 675–684.
33. Tepper, M. S. (2000). Sexuality and disability: The missing discourse of pleasure. *Sexuality and Disability, 18*(4), 283–290.
34. Novak, P. P., & Mitchell, M. M. (1988). Professional involvement in sexuality counseling for patients with spinal cord injuries. *The American Journal of Occupational Therapy, 42*(2), 105–112.
35. Chaves, E. S., Boninger, M. L., Cooper, R., Fitzgerald, S. G., Gray, D. B., & Cooper, R. A. (2004). Assessing the influence of wheelchair technology on perception of participation in spinal cord injury. *Archives of Physical Medicine and Rehabilitation, 85*(11), 1854–1858.
36. Barker, D. J., Reid, D., & Cott, C. (2004). Acceptance and meanings of wheelchair use in senior stroke survivors. *The American Journal of Occupational Therapy, 58*(2), 221–230.
37. Costa, V. S. P., Melo, M. R. A. C., Garanhani, M. L., & Fujisawa, D. S. (2010). Social representations of the wheelchair for people with spinal cord injury. *Revista Latino-Americana de Enfermagem, 18*(4), 755–762.
38. Rohmer, O., & Louvet, E. (2012). Implicit measures of the stereotype content associated with disability. *British Journal of Social Psychology, 51*(4), 732–740.
39. Gaete-Reyes, M. (2015). Citizenship and the embodied practice of wheelchair use. *Geoforum, 64*, 351–361.
40. Dickson, A., Allan, D., & O'carroll, R. (2008). Biographical disruption and the experience of loss following a spinal cord injury: An interpretative phenomenological analysis. *Psychology and Health, 23*(4), 407–425.

41. Barlew, L., Secrest, J., Guo, Z., Fell, N., & Haban, G. (2013). The experience of being grounded: A phenomenological study of living with a wheelchair. *Rehabilitation Nursing, 38*(4), 193–201.
42. Mann, W. C., Hurren, D., Charvat, B., & Tomita, M. (1996). Problems with wheelchairs experienced by frail elders. *Technology and Disability, 5*(1), 101–111.
43. Judd, F. K., Burrows, G. D., & Brown, D. J. (1986). Depression following acute spinal cord injury. *Spinal Cord, 24*(6), 358–363.
44. Klyce, D. W., Bombardier, C. H., Davis, T. J., Hartoonian, N., Hoffman, J. M., Fann, J. R., & Kalpakjian, C. Z. (2015). Distinguishing grief from depression during acute recovery from spinal cord injury. *Archives of Physical Medicine and Rehabilitation, 96*(8), 1419–1425.
45. Beedie, A., & Kennedy, P. (2002). Quality of social support predicts hopelessness and depression post spinal cord injury. *Journal of Clinical Psychology in Medical Settings, 9*(3), 227–234.
46. Cao, Y., Massaro, J. F., Krause, J. S., Chen, Y., & Devivo, M. J. (2014). Suicide mortality after spinal cord injury in the United States: Injury cohorts analysis. *Archives of Physical Medicine and Rehabilitation, 95*(2), 230–235.
47. Lohne, V. (2008). The battle between hoping and suffering: A conceptual model of hope within a context of spinal cord injury. *Advances in Nursing Science, 31*(3), 237–248.
48. Tutton, E., Seers, K., & Langstaff, D. (2009). An exploration of hope as a concept for nursing. *Journal of Orthopaedic Nursing, 13*(3), 119–127.
49. Littooij, E., Widdershoven, G. A., Stolwijk-Swüste, J. M., Doodeman, S., Leget, C. J., & Dekker, J. (2015). Global meaning in people with spinal cord injury: Content and changes. *The Journal of Spinal Cord Medicine., 39*(2), 197–205.
50. Tramonti, F., Gerini, A., & Stampacchia, G. (2015). Relationship quality and perceived social support in persons with spinal cord injury. *Spinal Cord, 53*(2), 120–124.
51. Monden, K. R., Trost, Z., Catalano, D., Garner, A. N., Symcox, J., Driver, S., Hamilton, G., & Warren, A. M. (2014). Resilience following spinal cord injury: A phenomenological view. *Spinal Cord, 52*(3), 197–201.
52. Wilson, C. S., Forchheimer, M., Heinemann, A. W., Warren, A. M., & McCullumsmith, C. (2017). Assessment of the relationship of spiritual well-being to depression and quality of life for persons with spinal cord injury. *Disability and Rehabilitation, 39*(5), 491–496.
53. Veith, E. M., Sherman, J. E., Pellino, T. A., & Yasui, N. Y. (2006). Qualitative analysis of the peer-mentoring relationship among individuals with spinal cord injury. *Rehabilitation Psychology, 51*(4), 289–298.
54. Dickson, A., Ward, R., O'Brien, G., Allan, D., & O'Carroll, R. (2011). Difficulties adjusting to post-discharge life following a spinal cord injury: An interpretative phenomenological analysis. *Psychology, Health and Medicine, 16*(4), 463–474.
55. Magasi, S., & Papadimitriou, C. (2022). Peer support interventions in physical medicine and rehabilitation: A framework to advance the field. *Archives of Physical Medicine and Rehabilitation, 103*(7), S222–S229.
56. Gassaway, J., Jones, M. L., Sweatman, W. M., Hong, M., Anziano, P., & DeVault, K. (2017). Effects of peer mentoring on self-efficacy and hospital readmission after inpatient rehabilitation of individuals with spinal cord injury: A randomized controlled trial. *Archives of Physical Medicine and Rehabilitation, 98*(8), 1526–1534.

Chapter 4
The Future

How do humans create identities? For some, it's their abilities; for others, it's the people in their lives; and for many, it is their ability to pursue a career and a dream. While all persons find this challenging, persons with spinal cord injuries have a greater burden with this pursuit. As discussed in Chap. 3, there are multiple losses that a person with a spinal cord injury (SCI) experiences beyond the actual physical change. This final chapter explores opportunities for education, avocation, and employment and identifies obstacles as well as prospects.

The initial SCI creates an alteration in every component of life. Research indicates that the initial 2–3 years is essential for development of identity and relearning how to function and live. Initially, attention is placed on understanding one's body and both relearning daily routines and creating new ones [1]. The focus of the persons with SCI is not on employment as much as wrapping their head around the changes they are experiencing.

The opportunity to participate in paid employment is positively associated with the quality of life and the adjustment following a spinal cord injury. Unfortunately, the more time that passes without a focus on pursuing employment opportunities, the harder it is to achieve employment [2]. Rates of employment are very low among persons with spinal cord injuries. There are several factors that play a role in pursuing employment. They include peer mentors, previous employment opportunities, and social supports. While it appears that there are little opportunities for this pursuit, there are in fact several organizations, foundations, and laws that exist to promote opportunity.

As previously explored in Chap. 3, many individuals with spinal cord injury experience a loss of sense of self and a separation from the world. This loss is physical and subjective. It encompasses the perception of one's body as well as one's capabilities. While in theory there should be nothing limiting access to the world for persons with disabilities, in reality there is plenty. Environmental and social barriers play a role in most aspects of everyday life, impacting all areas of one's daily routine. Society creates this disability. Thankfully, over time, there has been a greater

© The Author(s) 2022
J. Lieberman, *The Physical, Personal, and Social Impact of Spinal Cord Injury*,
SpringerBriefs in Public Health, https://doi.org/10.1007/978-3-031-18652-3_4

understanding of the impact of environmental barriers on the social world and on our ability to modify the environment to increase inclusion. This chapter examines the laws and acts that have been introduced over the years, as well as the programs that exist to promote increased opportunity for the persons with a spinal cord injury to live their best life. In this day and age, there is no reason for anyone to be denied access to education, employment, and socialization. There is still a large discrepancy between persons with and without disabilities in accessing employment and education and in achieving financial well-being. However, several laws have been drafted over the years to increase access to the world for this population.

4.1   Legislation

There are several bills and reforms that exist that have led to increased access to the world for all persons with disabilities. Persons with disabilities can credit the initial opportunity for inclusion to the Civil Rights movement.

4.1.1   Civil Rights and Access: From the Civil Rights Act to the ADA

Over the years, several legislative policies have been introduced to increase access for persons with disabilities and to promote engagement. For a very long time, persons with disabilities were denied basic human rights, which ultimately led to the introduction of these policies. Access today for persons with spinal cord injuries goes back to the 1960s Civil Rights movement, advanced farther in 1990 with the signing of the Americans with Disabilities Act and is still evolving today.

The Americans with Disabilities Act was born out of the desire of persons with disabilities to be active participants in the community, just like persons without disabilities. Individuals with disabilities wanted to be able to live their lives to the fullest and achieve the same desires and goals as everyone else. The predecessors to the ADA are the Civil Rights Act of 1964, the Rehabilitation Act of 1973, and the Education For All Handicapped Children Act of 1974, which has since been renamed the Individuals with Disabilities Education Act (IDEA).

The Civil Rights Act of 1964 was a product of the Civil Rights movement and the wave of unrest over discriminatory practices on all levels. The Civil Rights Act prohibited discrimination of public accommodations and federally funded programs on the basis of race, color, religion, sex, or national origin. Regardless of differences, the Civil Rights Act stated that no one will be victimized for being different. The Civil Rights Act also played a large role in the opportunity to vote and attend school as it reinforced the federal government's protection of voting rights and the desegregation of schools. It was inevitable that the Civil Rights movement would have led to the disability rights movement.

The Rehabilitation Act of 1973 (amended to the Act) is fundamentally a Civil Rights act focusing on individuals with disabilities. It prohibits discrimination in federally funded programs on the basis of disability. The Rehabilitation Act also focuses on improved access to social services, healthcare, recreation, housing, and transportation. There are several sections of this Act that are significant as they relate to the provision of services within the federal government, including sections 501, 503, and 508. Section 501 requires nondiscrimination in employment within the federal government and associated agencies. Section 503 prohibits discrimination among federal contractures. Section 508 requires that technology used by the federal government and associated agencies, both electronic and informational, be accessible for persons with disabilities. This is required for both employees and members of the general public.

Another key component to the Rehabilitation Act is that it encourages increased opportunity for educational access for persons with disabilities. One year after the Rehabilitation Act was introduced, the Education For All Handicapped Children Act was signed into law. This act focused on children's access and engagement, promoting mainstreaming education and the creation of an Individual Educational Plan (IEP). IDEA required that public schools provide education for children with disabilities in the least restrictive environment. It also required that the IEP be generated by a qualified special education team and that parents can request a fair hearing if they do not agree if their children are denied services.

Under the Americans with Disabilities Act, a person with a disability is identified as one with a physical or mental impairment that significantly limits one or more major life activities. The person with disability is someone who has a history of impairment or who is perceived by others as having an impairment.

The ADA is broken down into five categories or titles. The five titles under the ADA are Employment, State and Local Government Activities, Public Transportation, Public Accommodations, and Telecommunications Relay Services.

Title I requires that employers with 15 or more employees provide an equal opportunity for qualified individuals with disabilities. It obliges employers to provide all the benefits available to others and restricts questions regarding an applicant's disability prior to a job offer being made. Title I also requires that reasonable accommodations are provided to qualified individuals with disabilities, including physical or mental limitations, unless it results in undue hardship.

The concept of reasonable accommodations goes back to the 1970s and was written into regulations required by the Equal Employment Opportunity Commission (EEOC) and the Department of Justice. Some accommodations identified by the ADA are (Table 4.1) as follows:

Title II of the ADA requires that both state and local governments provide people with disabilities equal opportunity to benefit from all activities, services, and programs. Title II legally ensures that local and state governments are required to adhere to architectural standards when altering existing buildings or constructing new buildings. Additionally, for those buildings that cannot be modified, programs, services, and activities need to be moved to accessible buildings. This includes access to courts, voting sites, transportation, recreation, education, and

Table 4.1 Workplace accommodations

Making the workplace structurally accessible
Restructuring jobs to make best use of an individual's skill
Modifying work hours
Reassigning an employee with a disability to an equivalent position once available
Acquire/modify equipment/devices, materials, policies, and tests
Provide qualified readers for the blind or interpreters for the deaf

employment. Local governments must take action, unless these modifications to policies, practices, and procedures will result in financial or administrative burdens and alter the nature of the service, program, or activity being provided.

Title II also covers public transportation, including city buses, subways, commuter rail, and Amtrak. Title II states that transportation cannot discriminate against people with disabilities and that all newly purchased vehicles must be accessible, unless this would result in an undue burden. Under these circumstances paratransit, transportation for the handicapped, needs to be offered. This legislation was introduced in 1990 requiring that these changes be initiated, with several goals to be achieved over time. In 1993, key stations were required to be accessible, provided modifications did not create an undue burden. An extension was offered to trolley and commuter rail to 2010 and subway stations in 2020. While two thirds of stations are required to be accessible now, they are not. For example, in New York City alone, only 25% of the stations are accessible, with the goal of the Metropolitan Transportation Authority to achieve 95% station access by 2055.

In summary, Title II allows persons with disabilities the opportunity to access various areas of the world just like anyone else, through increased opportunities for access to buildings and transportation.

Title III prohibits discrimination in public accommodations operated by private entities. This includes not-for-profit and privately operated locations. The services provided include private transportation, restaurants, movie theaters, hotels, convention centers, retail stores, zoos, homeless shelters, day care facilities, fitness centers, sports arenas, and many more privately run commercial facilities. Effective 1992, entities that lease, rent, or own public accommodations cannot discriminate against persons with disabilities. They are prohibited from segregating or excluding others on the basis of disability. This includes reasonable modification to policy and practice, removal of environmental barriers, and making sure ancillary aids are available. Failure to provide these modifications and services is forbidden under Title III of the ADA. In addition, barriers that are present were required to be removed by 1992, provided it can be completed without difficulty or excessive expense.

Title III also covers professional, educational, and commercial buildings. All examinations, whether for academic purposes or vocational requirements, must be provided in a place that is accessible with accommodations and alternative provisions to address various needs. All commercial facilities must also comply with the architectural standards put in place by the ADA when performing new construction or modifications.

Titles II and III allow for access to all services, regardless of disability, by providing protection from discrimination due to disability. The planned outcome of enforcement of the combination of both Titles under the ADA is to ensure that most community environments and services that are available for persons without disabilities are accessible to persons with disabilities.

Title IV focuses on telecommunications and access for those with hearing and speech impairments. This includes telephone and television access. Title IV requires that all telephone companies establish relay services 24 hours a day, 7 days a week. Companies must provide technology or a third-party assistant to facilitate communication for those with hearing or speech impairments at all hours. Additionally, closed captioning is required for all public service announcements. Title IV was the predecessor to the Telecommunications Act of 1996, which required that all new technology and services be accessible. This includes televisions, cell phones, pagers, and telephones. This act required that accessible technology be available for all persons with disabilities. Because of the Telecommunications Act of 1996, all new television sets must include closed captioning.

4.1.2 Additional Legislation to Promote Access and Inclusivity

Other important acts, as they relate to persons with disabilities, are the Civil Rights of Institutionalized Persons Act, the Architectural Barriers Act, the Fair Housing Act, the Voting Accessibility for the Elderly and Handicapped Act of 1984, and the Voter Registration Act of 1993. These particular acts directly impact the ability for persons with disabilities to not only live in the community but to also be productive members of the society.

The Civil Rights of Institutionalized Persons Act allows the government to investigate institutions and their treatment of persons with disabilities. This includes, but is not limited to, nursing homes, psychiatric institutions, prisons, detention centers, and institutions for persons with developmental delays. This act allows for the initiation of an investigation and lawsuit when conditions are believed to be harmful. It promotes equal rights and humane treatment for those who are marginalized or not capable to defend themselves. For persons with SCI, this is an important legislation due to increased rates of nursing home admissions after discharge from acute rehabilitation.

The Architectural Barriers Act (ABA) was written and put into effect in 1968, more than 10 years prior to the ADA. It is the first Federal accessibility law. While the ADA introduced legally required modifications to private sector access, the ABA dealt specifically with the alteration and new design of buildings that are leased with federal funds.

The voting acts, including the Voting Accessibility for the Elderly and Handicapped Act and the Voter Registration Act, require that polling places be accessible and when they are not that alternative options are present for allowing for registration and voting, including aids and information. For the person with SCI, this guarantees the opportunity to vote, a right of all citizens. However, certain states have recently introduced laws that negatively impact access.

4.1.3 Advocacy

Advocacy for the person with SCI can be essential for recovery. Advocating for one's medical needs and for legislative change can provide persons with SCI control over both their body and their world. The persons with SCI however cannot advocate for themselves if they lack the knowledge of the primary and secondary conditions associated with their SCI. Education is an essential component of rehabilitation for functional progress and long-term health.

Self-advocacy is important for all persons with SCI due to the large number of healthcare providers lacking knowledge of complications associated with SCI. Research has shown that almost half of all primary care physicians and emergency department physicians are not aware of the signs or symptoms of the secondary conditions associated with SCI [3]. Lack of knowledge often leads to preventable complications. It therefore becomes important to have a good understanding of all components of SCI. Healthcare providers who do not specialize in SCI are often unaware of the multitude of risks and symptoms. Considerations for the person with SCI are the following:

- Requesting regular repositioning when in the ED to decrease incidence of pressure injury.
- Informing medical staff that fluctuations in blood pressure and heart rate can be signs of AD and should be treated accordingly.
- Due to impaired sensation, sensory response can be referred. Pain in one location may not indicate location of distress or injury.

Due to limited knowledge of the specific physiological changes to the system of the person with SCI, complications while receiving medical care are not uncommon. Pressure injury during hospitalization or emergency department stay is a frequently acquired hospital event [4]. Educating hospital personnel can decrease the incidence of these complications. Several advocacy organizations have created wallet cards identifying certain risk factors for persons with SCI, including pressure injury and AD.

Self-advocacy for legislative change is another area that the person with SCI should be exposed to. The person with SCI receives care, supplies, and equipment based upon legislation. Since these legislative changes can most directly impact them, the person with SCI becomes the ideal person to advocate for change. There are several independent organizations and coalitions of organizations that advocate for policy changes to ensure independence and inclusion. One such example is the Roll on Capitol Hill, a yearly advocacy event of United Spinal Association where hundreds of people with SCI and spinal cord disorders travel to Washington DC with their caretakers to meet with legislators and discuss issues that impact the quality of life, health, and independence of persons with SCI (Fig. 4.1).

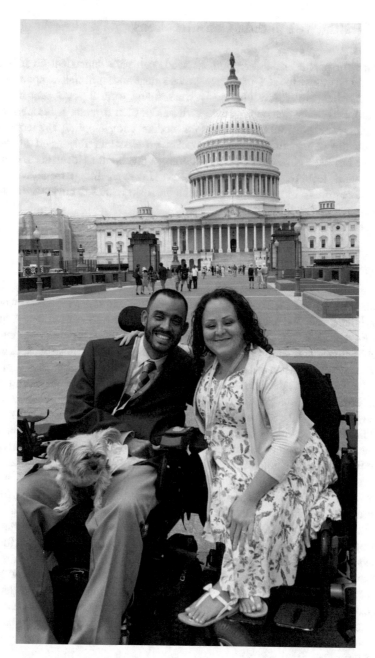

Fig. 4.1 Jose Hernandez and Jessica Delarosa; advocates

4.2   Healthcare Funding Considerations

Coverage for healthcare and equipment needs can vary dependent on individual funding. Persons with SCI can have private insurance through a spouse, their employer, Medicare if they previously worked and were 2 years post injury, or Medicaid. Private insurance coverage varies from plan to plan. It is important to know what your individual plan covers for medical care, supplies, and technology, including the explanation of out of pocket costs, deductibles, and allowable. Medicare has been covered in several sections in this book as it relates to complex rehabilitation technology and employment. However, for persons with SCI, Medicaid requires a more extensive examination as it relates to coverage of healthcare, support, and equipment.

4.2.1   Medicaid

An understanding of Medicaid is necessary to engage in a discussion on working and receiving benefits. Eligibility for Medicaid is based upon Modified Adjusted Gross Income (MAGI). This is used to determine eligibility for children, pregnant women, parents, and adults. While most states follow similar guidelines, there are state by state differences. It's important to check the eligible requirements of each state. Persons with disabilities are also eligible for Medicaid based upon MAGI. However, some person with SCI are eligible for Medicaid based on the income guidelines of the SSI program managed by the Social Security Administration.

Medicaid will provide personal care assistance in the home to help with bathing, dressing, eating, and other non-medical needs. The Affordable Care Act introduced the Community First Choice Option (CFCO), which provides additional care with activities of daily living and instrumental activities of daily living (IADL), including dressing, transfers, mobility, meal preparation, housekeeping, etc. This program also provides for health-related activities, including wound care and dressing changes. The goal of CFCO is to maintain persons in the community rather than requiring placement in a nursing home. The CFCO also provides the option for self-directed care and allows for selecting one's own caregiver. This allows for the opportunity to select friends or family to provide your ADL and IADL. Prior to this, these services were provided through the Home and Community Based Services waiver. Waivers are cap-based programs. This means that not everyone can enroll in the program. However, Medicaid is a need-based program so no one who requires Medicaid services should be denied. The CFCO ensured that those who qualified for these services received them.

Many persons with disabilities, including SCI, receive Medicaid benefits to cover not just hospitalization and medical needs but also services, equipment, and supplies. Medicaid will cover home attendant support based upon need. Medicaid will also cover supplies if they are determined to be medically necessary, including catheters, as well as complex rehabilitation technology and durable medical equipment, including wheelchairs, hospital beds, and equipment for the bathroom.

4.2.2 Crime Victims Fund

The Victims of Crimes Act (VOCA) was signed into law in 1984. This was established to provide federal support to local state programs that assist victims of federal or state crimes. The Office of Victims of Crime (OVC) was established in 1988 from an amendment to VOCA. OVC provides assistance and compensation. Assistance includes counseling, crisis support, shelter, criminal justice advocacy, and transportation. Compensation is provided through the Crime Victims Fund (The Fund), which the OVC oversees. The Fund receives a bulk of its money from criminal fines, forfeited bail, penalties, and other monies collected by the US Attorneys' Office, Federal Courts, and Federal Bureau of Prisons. Congress has also provided annual caps to ensure this fund does not run out.

14% of cases of SCI are a result of violence [5]. This violence is often in the form of sustaining a gunshot wound or from an assault. For persons with SCI who have received their injury from an act of violence, OVC and The Fund can provide lifetime support. The Fund can provide funding for CRT, covering equipment needs that are not reimbursed by insurance. Expenses covered include medical expenses, counseling, lost wages, and support. If the individual responsible for the crime is convicted, the person with SCI may be entitled to restitution.

The OVC consists of both national and local victim organizations. In order to qualify for support from OVC and The Fund, the person with SCI must report the crime to the police and cooperate with them as they work to solve the crime. They can apply for compensation through the local victim organization or online. However, once in the system, the resources can provide support throughout the life of the person with SCI.

4.3 Employment

Persons with SCI who are employed identify greater satisfaction with life, health, functional capabilities, and psychological adjustment [6]. Yet very few people with SCI are employed. There are several factors to this. This section explores some of the factors for such high rates of unemployment among persons with SCI.

4.3.1 Protections and Statistics

Employment protections are covered under the ADA. Under the ADA, it is unlawful to discriminate against a person with a disability. This includes but is not limited to employment agencies, labor organizations and labor management committees, state and local governments, and private employers. If you have a disability and are qualified to perform a job duty, you cannot be discriminated against due to that disability. Furthermore, the ADA provides protections whether you have a history of disability or your employer believes you have a disability, even if you don't. These discriminations carry over to recruitment, hiring, training, job assignment, pay, benefits, promotions, firing, and any other employment-related activity.

It is important to know that an employer cannot ask you if you are disabled, cannot require you to take a medical examination, and cannot ask you the nature of your disability. They are able to ask what reasonable accommodation is required for you to be able to perform your duties. But, they are not allowed to require a medical examination unless it is something that all employees must undergo. Furthermore, if that examination provides indication of a disability, they are not allowed to refuse your hiring or fire you because of it.

In order to fall under these protections, there must be documented history of a disability or a perception of a disability. You must also be qualified to perform the required duties and/or essential functions of the job. This is with or without reasonable accommodation. A reasonable accommodation is any modification to a job or work environment that allows the qualified person with a disability to perform their job duties and enjoy the benefits of employment as those without disabilities do. Some of the possible accommodations are as follows (Table 4.2):

Protection from discrimination falls under the US Equal Employment Opportunity Commission (EEOC). It is the EEOC that enforces federal laws making it illegal to discriminate against an employee on the basis of race, color, age, gender identity, religion national origin, and disability. Under the EEOC, if discrimination has occurred, a job discrimination lawsuit can be filed. The EEOC will complete a thorough investigation to determine if in fact discrimination has occurred and will file a lawsuit if it is determined to be a legitimate case of discrimination. There are however several considerations, including employer, number of employees, type of discrimination, etc. It is important to know your rights before attempting to sue on the basis of disability discrimination. To determine this, it is helpful to review information provided by EEOC.

The Office of Disability Employment Policy (ODEP) began in 2001 as part of the department of labor. ODEP is a federally funded organization that promotes policy to increase success in the workplace for persons with disabilities. The goal of ODEP is to provide initiatives to promote employment for persons with disabilities through the development of policy and grants and by eliminating barriers. The aim of ODEP is to ensure that persons with disabilities have unlimited employment opportunities. On their website, ODEP tracks numerous statistics, including employment and unemployment rates among persons with and without disabilities.

Table 4.2 Employment accommodations

Modification to equipment or devices
Modified work schedules
Providing an interpreter or reader
Restructuring the job
Adjusting policies and training materials

The most recent numbers posted are staggering. While the rate has changed over time, the discrepancy between persons with and without disabilities and their employment status is vast.

In 2019, 33.6% of the persons with disabilities and 77.3% of the persons without disabilities between the ages of 16 and 64 made up the labor force, whereas only 8% of the persons with disabilities and 3.6% of the persons without disabilities were unemployed. In March 2021, 20.2% of the persons with disabilities and 66.8% of the persons without disabilities between the ages of 16 and 64 made up the labor force, whereas 12.2% of the persons with disabilities and 6.5% of the persons without disabilities were unemployed. Of note, the rate of unemployment and job loss from 2020 to 2021 increased due to COVID (Population Survey, Bureau of Labor Statistics). While both populations decreased in workforce participation, the percentage of persons with disabilities who are unemployed is greater. While the Department of Labor, ODEP, and other organizations have worked hard to decrease these numbers, there are several other factors at play. This includes the opportunity to continue to receive benefits.

4.3.2 Working and Receiving Benefits

Persons with SCI require ongoing care and supplies to maintain their health. These needs often outweigh those of the non-SCI population. Healthcare benefits are therefore essential for the person with SCI even once fully employed. However most private insurance plans do not cover basic needs, including supplies and caretakers. This is one of the primary factors that fewer persons with disabilities are actively employed. In order to purse gainful employment, the person with SCI often requires additional or alternative funding to manage their health.

4.3.2.1 Medicaid

Legislation exists to facilitate living in the community, pursuit of education, and employment. How this translates to real life is a challenge. There are certain barriers that exist to achieving this level of independence. A primary factor impacting the ability to live one's best life is finances. In order to receive benefits for medical and rehabilitation intervention and supplies, the individual cannot have a monthly income above a certain value. In most states, that is less than $1500 per month and less than $18,000 a year. An individual with an income above this can still acquire Medicaid, but there is a cost to this. Section 1902(a)(17) of the Social Security Act allows for a Medical Spend Down, also known as the Medicaid Excess Program. Under the Spend Down, if there is too much income, called excess income, this excess can be paid off in order to receive Medicaid to cover medical expenses. This excess is used to pay for medical bills. If your medical expenses are higher than the excess income you are receiving, you can still receive your Medicaid benefits. You would just pay a portion of the bill monthly and Medicaid would cover the rest. For example, if an individual with SCI has an income $100 over the allowable, once they pay $100 into the medical bill, the remainder would be covered by Medicaid. Medical expenses can include but are not limited to medical bills, transportation, equipment, including wheelchairs, prosthetics, hearing aids and glasses, and prescription drugs.

4.3.2.2   Pooled Trust

The second option is a pooled trust. The Omnibus Budget Reconciliation Act of 1993 (OBRA '93) allows persons with disabilities to set up trusts to manage excess funds while still qualifying for Medicaid. This act was extended in 1999 when the Ticket to Work and Work Incentives Improvement Act of 1999 (P.L. 106–170) was passed to ensure this program would continue within the SSI program. Pooled trusts are the most common form, where resources of multiple persons with disabilities are combined. This results in a larger overall amount of capital to invest. These trusts are usually established and managed by a non-profit organization, which often also serves as the trustee or co-trustee. Each individual pays into the trust and receives income based upon their share of the entire trust. Oftentimes, it is the excess income that is paid into the trust (the excess income from the Spend Down). When this excess income is deposited into the pooled trust, the funds remain available for paying bills. For example, the trust can be used to set up automatic payments for recurring bills such as rent and other monthly bills. The funds cannot be withdrawn as cash but can be submitted to cover various regularly occurring costs.

4.4   Employment Programs

There are programs that exist to facilitate return to work and employment opportunities. These provide assessment of skill and training for new opportunities as well as funding to ensure management of healthcare complications related to SCI.

4.4.1   The Ticket to Work and Work Incentives Improvement Act of 1999 (P.L. 106–170)

Individuals who have previously contributed to Social Security through employment can qualify for Social Security benefits. The Social Security Administration (SSA) provides disability benefits under two programs: Social Security Disability Insurance (SSDI) and Social Security Income (SSI). Funding for these programs comes from either SSA (SSDI) or the Federal Government (SSI). SSDI funding comes from the Social Security Trust fund. The amount of money one receives from this is based upon the individual's earnings or that of one's spouse, parents, etc.

A person with SSDI can qualify for Medicare benefits after 24 months since the onset of the disability. Qualifications for Medicare are being over the age of 65, having end-stage renal disease, or being under the age of 65 and having a disability. As stated in the previous section, persons with disabilities qualify for Medicaid based upon income, with options to spend down. Persons with SSDI qualify for Medicare based upon how much money they made when employed or how much their spouse or parents made. The needs of the person with SCI are extensive. In Chap. 1, multiple secondary complications were examined. Treatment for these can be costly, making emergent medical coverage essential.

One of the important pieces to the Ticket to Work and Work Incentives Improvement Act of 1999 for SSDI beneficiaries was the inclusion of extended Medicare Part A coverage for a total of 93 consecutive months. This ensured that if a person with SCI required inpatient hospitalization due to, for example, a pressure injury or sepsis from a UTI, they can travel to the hospital and be admitted to the medicine unit and their Medicare Part A will cover the cost. While this will not cover the cost of seeing a physician in their private office (that is covered under Part B), it will cover inpatient hospitalization, ensuring availability of urgent medical care.

4.4.2 Vocational Rehabilitation

For persons who have had a dramatic change in their life, like a spinal cord injury, and need to explore other avenues for employment, Vocational Rehabilitation (VR) is an option. On June 2, 1920, President Woodrow Wilson signed into law the National Civilian Vocational Rehabilitation Act (Smith-Fess Act of 1920). This opened the door to the State Vocational Rehabilitation Services Program, which was authorized by the Rehabilitation Act. This program provides grants to states for VR programs that provide funding for training individuals with disabilities. Training consists of preparing the individual with a disability for competitive integrated employment so they can achieve a level of economic independence. Programs are created to identify the strengths and weakness of each client and to help them capitalize on their skills to achieve and maintain employment.

VR counselors evaluate the person with SCI to determine their limitations, skills, interests, previous abilities, and barriers to employment. The assessment process can include either simulation or actual performance. Due to their extensive experience working with persons with SCI, the VR counselor will often work closely with the individual and their employer to assist with accommodations and job site modifications once employment is acquired.

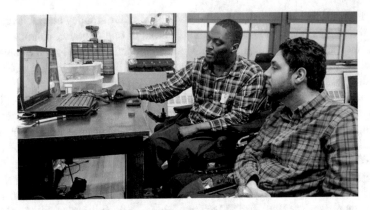

Fig. 4.2   Stefan Henry and Eli Ramos, Level the Curve Designs

4.4.3   Employment Barriers and Opportunities

Persons with SCI can be capable of anything. The opportunities for employment are extensive, particularly with today's technology and the ability to work around one's disability. There are however certain barriers to achieving employment. Transportation is one of the leading barriers [7]. Additional barriers include accessibility, health and physical limitations, and workplace discrimination. Early education of the potential barriers increases the opportunities for success in pursuing employment.

Telework can increase inclusion of persons with SCI into the workforce. The COVID pandemic made working from home more acceptable, increasing opportunities for employment for persons with disabilities [8]. There are industries and avenues being developed daily for persons with SCI to pursue employment. Engineering has been frequently pursued as an opportunity to create adaptive devices and CRT for persons with varying impairments, including SCI. Through personal experience, the engineer with SCI is best able to identify the needs of the population of people with SCI (Fig. 4.2).

A new area garnering attention is the hospitality industry, due in large part to the increased exposure of certain persons with SCI to the general population. Identifying the possibilities for easy environmental modifications and adaptations has led to new opportunities for both employment and ownership (Fig. 4.3).

4.5   Living in the Community

Another important role of the Rehabilitation Services Act is to provide funding for independent living programs. Centers for independent living provide resources and supports to individuals with disabilities to facilitate integration into the community. Under Title VII, Chap. 1 of the Rehabilitation Act, the purpose of independent living programs is to create an environment of consumer support, self-help and

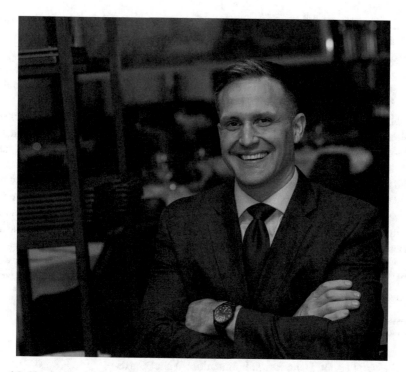

Fig. 4.3 Yannick Benjamin, sommelier, restauranteur, and business owner

self-determination, advocacy, peer mentorship, and equal access for increased inclusion of persons with disabilities into mainstream society. Centers for independent living encourage independence, empowerment, leadership, and productivity to enable persons with disabilities to become active participants with the world.

In the 1960s, as the Civil Rights Movement was growing, more and more individuals with disabilities were leaving institutions and moving into the community. This is where the birthplace of the Independent Living Movement came from. Centers for Independent Living are consumer controlled. They are community based and operated by persons with disabilities to provide peer support, information, advocacy, living skills training, and transition. The concept was that persons with disabilities have a greater awareness of the needs of persons with disabilities. Funding for Centers for Independent Living is provided to the state based upon the States Plan for Independent Living (SPIL), which is a 3-year plan of what services are provided. The National Council of Independent Living data identifies that there are currently approximately 403 Centers for Independent Living with 330 branch offices and 56 Statewide Independent Living Councils. Given the numbers of persons with SCI who lack proper housing, this number is unfortunately quite low.

The Medicaid Home and Community Based Service (HCBS) Waiver Program for persons with SCI was established in 1981. The goal of the waiver program was to decrease cost of care for persons with SCI by moving them out of institutions and nursing homes and into the community. The waiver program provides some funding for residential, nursing, home health, respite care, and case management. Research has identified that the cost is significantly less to house people in the community [9]. Unfortunately, there are a large number of states with waiting lists, resulting in person's with SCI having to remain in institutions for longer periods of time. However, for those persons with SCI who lack accessible housing, this is a good opportunity to attempt to access accessible housing.

The 1999 Olmstead v. L.C. decision by the Supreme Court ruled that states are obligated to meet the needs of persons with disabilities in accordance with the ADA. This decision led to integrated housing, employment, transportation, and community services for persons with disabilities. The mandate requires persons with disabilities have access to community-based living settings in order to live fully integrated lives. Under Olmstead v. L.C., waiting lists can remain, but they need to move along at a faster rate. Unfortunately, the Supreme Court did not identify a rate of time for waiting lists. In a Medicaid and CHIP Payment and Access Commission report from 2017, the average wait throughout the states was 2 1/2 years.

Programs exist for community living and integration for persons with SCI. However, many of these programs vary from state to state. For more information on what your state offers, refer to the local agency's website.

Resources
- United Spinal Association
  unitedspinal.org
- Christopher and Dana Reeve Foundation: Wallet Cards
  christopherreeve.org
- Job Accommodation Network
  askjan.org
- disABLEDperson Inc., Jobs for Disabled
  disabledperson.com
- HEATH Resource Center at the National Youth Transitions Center (National Clearinghouse on Postsecondary Education for Individual with Disabilities)
  heath.gwu.edu
- Office of Victims of Crime
  ovc.org
- Equal Employment Opportunity Commission
  eeoc.gov
- Statewide Independent Living Councils
  ncil.org
- Medicaid and CHIP Payment and Access Commission
  macpac.gov
- Government Benefits
  usa.gov/benefits
- Administration for Community Living
  acl.gov
- Independent Living Research Utilization
  ilru.org

References

1. Hilton, G., Unsworth, C., & Murphy, G. (2018). The experience of attempting to return to work following spinal cord injury: A systematic review of the qualitative literature, disability and rehabilitation. *Disability and Rehabilitation, 40*(15), 1745–1753.
2. Hammel, J. (1999). The life rope: A transactional approach to exploring worker and life role development. *Work, 12*, 47–60.
3. Houlihan, B., Brody, M., Plant, A., Skeels, S. E., Zazula, J., Pernigotti, D., et al. (2016). Health care self-advocacy strategies for negotiating health care environments: Analysis of recommendations by satisfied consumers with SCI and SCI practitioners. *Topics in Spinal Cord Injury Rehabilitation, 22*(1), 13–26.
4. Van der Wielen, H., Post, M. W. M., Lay, V., Gläsche, K., & Scheel-Sailer, A. (2016). Hospital-acquired pressure ulcers in spinal cord injured patients: Time to occur, time until closure and risk factors. *Spinal Cord, 54*(9), 726–731.
5. Spinal cord injury facts and figures at a glance: 2018 SCI data sheet. University of Alabama at Birmingham National Spinal Cord Injury Statistical Center.
6. Bryce, T. N., Huang, V., & Escalon, M. X. (2021). Spinal cord injury. In *Braddom's physical medicine and rehabilitation* (pp. 1049–1100). Elsevier.
7. Lidal, I. B., Huynh, T. K., & Biering-Sørensen, F. (2007). Return to work following spinal cord injury: A review. *Disability and Rehabilitation, 29*(17), 1341–1375.
8. Schur, L. A., Ameri, M., & Kruse, D. (2020). Telework after COVID: A "silver lining" for workers with disabilities? *Journal of Occupational Rehabilitation, 30*(4), 521–536.
9. Kitchener, M., Ng, T., & Harrington, C. (2004). Medicaid 1915 (c) home and community-based services waivers: A national survey of eligibility criteria, caps, and waiting lists. *Home Health Care Services Quarterly, 23*(2), 55–69.

Index

© The Author(s) 2022
J. Lieberman, *The Physical, Personal, and Social Impact of Spinal Cord Injury*,
SpringerBriefs in Public Health, https://doi.org/10.1007/978-3-031-18652-3